Hot Nursing Careers for the 21st Century

Hot Nursing Careers for the 21st Century

111 Frequently Asked Questions About Entering Nursing

A Practical Guide for New or Seasoned Nurses

Micheline D. Birger

iUniverse, Inc.
New York   Bloomington   Shanghai

Hot Nursing Careers for the 21st Century
111 Frequently Asked Questions About Entering Nursing

iUniverse books may be ordered through booksellers or by contacting:

iUniverse
1663 Liberty Drive
Bloomington, IN 47403
www.iuniverse.com
1-800-Authors (1-800-288-4677)

Because of the dynamic nature of the Internet, any Web addresses or links contained in this book may have changed since publication and may no longer be valid.

The information, ideas, and suggestions in this book are not intended as a substitute for professional medical advice. Before following any suggestions contained in this book, you should consult your personal physician. Neither the author nor the publisher shall be liable or responsible for any loss or damage allegedly arising as a consequence of your use or application of any information or suggestions in this book.

ISBN: 978-0-595-48852-0 (pbk)
ISBN: 978-0-595-60870-6 (ebk)

Printed in the United States of America

Contents

Introduction/Bio of Micheline

I wrote this book to educate, entertain and enlighten anybody who chooses to look at the nursing profession as a job, a career choice, or simply wants the education and the knowledge that it provides. This is especially true in today's health care climate where consumers are overwhelmed with "the system". Today's customer is oversaturated with health care information. Having health knowledge in this new millennium is imperative. A basic nursing education can help one to "untangle the weeds" about what is the best choice for their personal healing and/or their loved ones as well as serving their community at large, wherever that may be.

I am an **RN, BSN**. In English, that means I am a Registered Nurse with a ***Bachelors of Science in Nursing***. Quite frankly, I do not know whether I am bragging or complaining. Either way, it is simply a statement of fact. I hold a degree from the ***University of Maryland*** in Baltimore, Maryland. USA. I have had my **RN** since 1972. I went step by step through the ranks. I started off as a candy-striper in high school and then I became an **LPN** at 19. I then entered an Associate Degree program and graduated from the ***Community College of Baltimore*** in 1972 with an **ADN**. (*Associates Degree in Nursing*)

I have, to this date, 2008, almost 36 years of experience in the profession. I have worked in New York, California, Iowa, Maryland, and New Jersey. In short, nationally. It really doesn't matter where I have worked. One truth remains constant. Health care in this country, at this pivotal time in history, is in crisis. It is a real mess. We have the technology. We have the hard science. We have so much wonderful knowledge; yet with all of this research and information the state of health care or the lack thereof is super dysfunctional in the USA. "But doc I got this pain and it won't go away, it's called who shall pay? Who shall pay?" Modern medicine in America-heal thyself! Heal the dysfunctional health delivery system in the US of A.

The only reason I went to nursing school is because my mother wanted me to. I always wanted to be a writer. I wanted to write for ***National Geographic*** and travel on assignment to exotic places. But, in my efforts to please my mother, that never manifested-yet. She wanted me to marry a doctor. That didn't happen either. I am not saying that it could or could not happen. It doesn't really matter to me anymore. I am more in love with my writing, which is my truth.

In my early years of nursing, I worked in university hospitals in Baltimore, Maryland. I worked in Adult Neurology and Neurosurgery and in the Post-Anesthetic Recovery Room. I also worked in Pediatric Neurology and Neurosurgery.

While I was at the **University of Maryland** in the 1970's, sometimes I would work in the ER if I wasn't busy at night in the Recovery Room. Never a dull moment in the ER, that's for sure. I drifted between **University of Maryland** and **Johns Hopkins Hospitals** in the 70's. Never a dull moment in those daze. Experience, I received world-class experience in those institutions.

After I got my solid experience and degree in nursing from the East, I went West. California was my home for almost 20 years. I mostly freelanced my skills through nursing agencies in San Francisco. I love the Bay Area. I was able to do many disciplines in nursing. ICU; CCU; PICU; psychiatry-both adult and child; general pediatrics and occasionally general floor nursing. While I was in San Francisco I started my own small business of providing emergency management to corporations having conventions in town. I also did many types of eclectic jobs such as insurance reviews and medical reviews. One of the Bay Area Corporations even sent me down to Mexico!

Before I left Maryland, I also moonlighted in two prisons; worked in a Job Corps Center for disadvantaged youths; worked at an Evangelical Gathering for 5000 people; worked at construction sites; and even did ear piercing in department stores all through an agency. I even marketed for a home health agency to hospitals.

As a hobby in San Francisco, I started doing improvisational comedy in the early eighties. I would come home feeling good all the time after performing. I wondered what was wrong with me because I felt so good after I laughed. At that time, the whole laughter and health movement was beginning to gain mainstream popularity. Norman Cousins famous book **Anatomy of an Illness** was on the *New York Times* bestseller list for a very long time. In his book, he chronicled his journey with a degenerative disease called "ankylosing spondylitis". In his book he talks on how he healed himself of the disease utilizing mega doses of Vitamin C and hard laughter. He reversed his illness in a period of about six months. Laughter was his medicine, his therapy. He then went from writing for the *Saturday Evening Post* to Professor Emeritus at **UCLA Medical School.**

I then put together my own seminar series called **Health as Humor: Humor as Health.** Or more aptly put, the **HAH: HAH Workshops**. I then became a public lecturer as well as a seminar leader. I taught nurses for continuing education units on the value of laughter on health and well-being. I even had some physicians come to my workshops for nurses. Now, that's a switch. I gave public lectures at the *University of California*; the *Safeway Corporation*; *the Whole Life Expo's* in San Francisco and Los Angeles; *Kaiser Hospital* in San Francisco as well as countless other organizations in the San Francisco Bay Area. I also spoke on numerous radio shows on the topic. *All of this attention because I was a nurse who spoke on laughter* *and health.* It all started with a flyer that I hung up in San Francisco Hospitals about health and humor. Go figure.

By this time I had evolved into doing some stand-up comedy—jest for the Zen of it—in San Francisco open mike comedy clubs. I hung out with comics. I also hung out with a group of nurses called *Nurses in Transition* in San Francisco. They were very much into alternative health; metaphysical and spiritual healing as well as herbs; chiropractic medicine; visualization; naturopathic as well as other natural healing modalities. They taught me that healing is a personal issue. It is up to the consumer of modern day health care to do their due diligence in finding what the best treatment for their own personal healing. Some treatments, works across the board, other treatments are more individual. It is up to the person to find out what works for them.

I wrote a manuscript called **Health as Humor: Humor as Health** or the **HAH! HAH! Book.** I interviewed tons of people for the book. This was the mid-eighties. I did have an excerpt published in a professional nurse's publication called **California Nursing Today.** I believe this was around 1985–86. The article was called *Is Laughter the Best Medicine?* I remember that I sent a copy to Norman Cousins in Los Angeles. He acknowledged the article and wrote me a nice note back to me on **UCLA** stationery. I will be publishing that book at sometime in the near future. Interesting, here it has been more than 20 years since the subject was first made accepted and here it is undergoing another renaissance. Why? I think because we need to hear the message again, and again and again. Especially now with the whole world situation and the US being in such chaos again.

I have always been deeply interested in how the brain works. We know so much yet we know so little. I worked in the discipline of psychiatry in the mid-nineties in one of the premier psych hospitals on the East Coast. I lead psychiatric groups throughout the day. I also worked in general psychiatry and child and adolescent psychiatry. I also went to the *dissociative unit* on occasion if they asked me to. Remember the movie, **The Three Faces of Eve**? Remember all of her multiple personalities? I witnessed some clients have 16 personalities. The mind can be so strong yet so fragile at the same time. After I got this solid experience on the East Coast, I went back to the West Coast and worked in acute care psychiatry in San Francisco. I then started doing travel contracts and just worked in psychiatry exclusively.

It is fascinating to watch some of the psychiatric meds take effect on acutely ill patients. It is interesting to observe the psych diagnoses and their different behavioral manifestations. More intriguing is how people respond to stress in their lives. It is also interesting to observe how people consciously or unconsciously choose to heal or not. But, back to the purpose of this book. The purpose of this book is to see if the nursing profession is something that you think you may want to pursue or you are a nurse and you are looking to expand your scope.

Regardless what one chooses to do in life, everything is an educational process. I even taught nurse's aides for their state certification. Very basic. Very simple. I even worked in Long Term Care as the psychiatric nurse for the facility. My soul prefers writing and lecturing.

I decided to make this book simple and easy. **Questions & Answers**. In everything that you do in life, remember to follow your heart and your intuition. Knowledge is power. Happy career choices to you!

I Am

Micheline

1. Is Nursing a calling?

A *calling?* Depends on who's asking. If you are seeing a shrink for whatever reasons, and you tell him or her that you are "hearing voices", that may or may not be such a hot idea that you are "hearing voices" but on a more serious note … a deeper sense … a *calling?* I think probably that it is. I believe that we need to heed that little voice that echoes louder and louder within us in order to propel us to action. Action in the direction that is most in tune with our *inner calling.*

A lot of folks enter the profession because they want to help people. Serving people comes in many shapes and forms … so is it a *calling?* Or is it a stable job with benefits? I say follow your passion, follow your bliss. There are countless ways to make a living. A *calling?* That is a tough call … but of course Joan of Arc did have a *calling,* didn't she?

2. What is the difference between a nurse's aide; a practical/vocational nurse and a registered nurse?

Education, education, education. A *Nurse's Aide* usually has to be certified in the state where they live. They must go through approximately 80-100 hours of classroom theory/training. They usually have simple classes in anatomy and physiology; medical terminology; diseases; legal implications and other technical knowledge. Depending on the environment where they choose to work, they are trained further in that area.

Upon satisfactory completion of the bookwork education, they then must complete 40 hours of clinical work. (Usually this is in a nursing home under the supervision of a registered nurse) When they have completed this satisfactorily, then they are eligible to graduate.

There are many schools that offer this training. Technical institutes, community colleges and some nursing homes teach this skill. Upon satisfactory completion of this course program, they are then certified and registered within the state of origin. (Varies from state to state) After a period of approximately four months after graduation and solid work experience, the nurse's aide is then eligible to take the state *Geriatric Nurse's Aide Exam.* (Again, varies from state to state) Successful completion of this exam usually means a higher hourly salary level. Nurse's aides are not allowed to give medications. They are not a nurse. They may not say that they are. That is misrepresentation.

A *LVN* (licensed vocational nurse) or an *LPN* (licensed practical nurse) is a person who has satisfactorily completed either one year or one and a half years of technical training. After graduation, they are eligible to take the state examination in order to be licensed. They are able to give medications. In some places, they are also able to give IV (intravenous) medications after proper certification(s). They can do some tasks such as insert a catheter into the bladder of a male or female patient. They can plan, implement and evaluate care delivered. They usually work under the supervision of a *Registered Nurse*.

A *Registered Nurse, RN*, is an individual who has completed a two, three or four year nursing program. They supervise Nurse's Aides, Licensed Practical Nurses/Vocational Nurses. They are licensed by the *State Board of Nursing*. They can further their education and enter into a variety of specialty fields. This would include but not limited to: nurse anesthetist; nurse psychotherapist; nurse practitioner; forensic nursing or a masters trained clinical specialists in a variety of areas. They can manage facilities; hospital units; teach; write; their scope is defined by the *Nurse Practice Act* for their particular specialty and their governing state rules/regulations.

3. Do I have to go to college to be a nurse?

Since the three year nursing programs have virtually faded out, the answer is yes. Depending on the individual's situation, many nursing candidates elect to go to a two year associate's degree program. This is a comprehensive program. It is usually given at community colleges. Upon completion of the program, the graduates are then eligible to take the state board for licensure as a registered nurse. Many people choose to take a two year program and take their boards. They are then registered nurses. Many nurses then continue their education and pursue higher degrees.

Many nurses go to four year universities and/or colleges. They take many liberal arts classes in addition to their science and math courses. *John Hopkins School of Nursing* offers an accelerated program of 13 months to folks who already have a college degree in another discipline.

4. What kind of courses will they make me take for a *Registered Nurse*?

That depends on where you go to school and what the requirements are. Usually two semesters in Anatomy and Physiology are required. Microbiology, Chemistry, Nutrition, Mathematics, Humanities, English and Psychology are usually other requirements. Once one is accepted into the nursing curriculum, then they must take all of the nursing courses as outlined by the school.

Once again, the course structure is different depending on whether one goes to a two or four year program. No matter what a future nurse may decide to do, to go to a two or a four year program, the state board exam will be the same. This is all dependent on satisfactory completion of the program.

When I took my RN boards in 1972 in Maryland, I was tested in Medical; Surgical; Maternal and Child Health; Pediatrics and Psychiatry. I believe at that time it took two days to complete. Each state has its own rules and regulations on giving the test to prospective nurses.

5. Isn't nursing physically hard?

Yes, yes it is. Hospital and long-term care can be physically grueling and exhausting. Most employers expect new nurses to have at least one year of Medical-Surgical experience before they consider them for other health care opportunities. The expectation is that new nurses must have a rock solid foundation of general hospital experience in order to qualify for other areas of health care.

6. Suppose I don't want to work in a hospital, what other places can I work in as a nurse?

That depends on the individual nurse and what their specific qualifications are. For example, suppose a nurse has a background in sales. He/she could be hired to market pharmaceuticals and medical supplies. Usually the employers will put them through their own training program for the particular product that they are marketing/selling.

If the nurse has a background in the written word, they may be hired for medical editing or medical journalism. A nurse may have a computer background. They could be hired as consultants in planning medical information technology. A nurse may also work with lawyers or do chart reviews for insurance companies. Once again, usually this requires solid hospital experience.

Generally, if a new nurse wants to work in an alternative setting such as a clinic or doctor's office, the one year of solid hospital experience generally applies. Again, this is a highly individual process. Each potential employer will evaluate the specific skills of the nurse.

7. What is the difference between an ICU; CCU; PICU; SICU and NICU?

Generally speaking, an *ICU-Intensive Care Unit* is a specialized unit where patients are in need of constant monitoring/care. They are usually critically ill. Sometimes they are combined with *Surgical Intensive Care Units.*

In general, a patient who is in an *Intensive Care Unit* has tons of very expensive and sophisticated equipment in and around them. The patient is usually quite ill. Usually the nurse has one or two patients in an *ICU.*

A *CCU-Coronary Care Unit* is an intensive care unit that usually specializes in heart conditions such as heart attacks or heart blockages, etc. The patient is attached to a heart monitor. They must be observed closely to see how their condition progresses, either good or bad. They are usually considered acutely ill and are treated accordingly.

A *PICU-Pediatric Intensive Care Unit* is an intensive care unit that specializes in children. Usually, the age group is infancy to 18 years of age. Common reasons why children are in intensive care units are for breathing problems and/or accidents. Of course there are many other reasons such as certain surgeries or other medical conditions that require constant monitoring. Children's conditions can change extremely rapidly and they must be observed accordingly.

A *NICU-Newborn Intensive Care Unit* is where premature babies and high-risk newborns are taken care of. Some premature babies stay in the *NICU* for months after they are born because they have breathing and feeding difficulties. High-risk newborns are usually babies with birth deformities or other extraordinary medical complications after birth.

8. What kind of money will I make as a nurse?

That's a good question. It depends on location, location, location. Initially, in order to entice new graduates to hospitals, hospitals offer high starting salaries for new grads. If a nurse decides to stay in a particular facility then they would receive yearly increments or cost of living increases. Places like New York City and San Francisco pay nurses more but the cost of living is much higher than other areas of the USA.

Generally speaking (and this is subject to change in a heartbeat and a sneeze in health care), the Southern States pay less. The best way to find out is to look on the Internet and do a search under *Career Builders* or some other job search engine. But, no matter which way you cut, dice or splice it, you can make a living as a nurse. If you want to get rich as a nurse, write a best-selling book, win the lottery or have a relative who is a savvy investment whiz show you how to leverage your hard-earned money.

9. What is a psychiatric nurse?

A psychiatric nurse is a registered nurse who works with the mentally ill. He/she may work in a general hospital in an inpatient psychiatric unit. He/she may do emergency room assessments. Some psychiatric nurses work for insurance companies; run psychiatric groups; work in prisons or work in specialty psychiatric hospitals. Some psych nurses concentrate in children and adolescents. Some work with substance abuse and addiction issues. Some work with eating disorders. Some work with geriatric clients. I once worked in Manhattan in a methadone clinic on a travel contract.

Some psychiatric nurses require further certification. For example, a nurse may choose to be a nurse-psychotherapist. She is able to work independently but is not allowed to prescribe psychiatric medications. She may recommend to the supervising psychiatrist medications but it is up to the Medical Doctor to prescribe the medications. Many universities have *Psychiatric Nurse Practitioner* programs. The advanced practice nurse usually works as part of a mental health team under the umbrella of a board-certified psychiatrist. www.nursesource.org/psychiatric.html or www.apna.org is two websites for further information.

10. What is a hospice?

A hospice is a specialized wing in a nursing home; a dedicated branch in a hospital or a separate facility where patients who are terminally ill decide to go to have a peaceful death. Comfort measures such as pain medications and a non-hospital home-like setting assist these clients make the transition. Round the clock nursing care is provided for these patients. We will expand on this towards the end of this book.

11. How come nurses have to work all hours?

Another good question. In a nutshell, nurses have to work all hours because people get sick 24 hours a day, seven days a week. Hospitals, nursing homes and other facilities have the obligation to insure the public that their loved ones are taken care of 24/7.

12. Can I set up my own shingle as a nurse?

That really depends on the state that the nurse lives in and what specialty they have. For example, a nurse anesthetist may build up a practice by working with private physicians who do the surgery in their office(s). This is usually in an *In and out Surgery Center(s)*, (Ambulatory Care Surgical Centers) or plastic surgery offices. The nurse anesthetist is able to work in different offices during the week.

Laws are always changing in different states. In general, in order for a nurse to set out her own shingle as a health care practitioner she needs further education in addition to the standard RN. Of course there are always exceptions to the rule and some nurses are extremely business savvy. They are nurses who start their own agencies. These agencies supply nurses to hospitals, nursing homes and other types of health care facilities.

Some nurse entrepreneurs go into legal nurse consulting or other health-related businesses where their technical knowledge is a strong asset in promoting their own businesses.

13. What is the advantage to going to nursing school rather than medical school?

Another excellent question. It all boils down to the individual and whether they want to or not put in the extra years of education and study in order to become a doctor. Some nurses go into the nursing profession in order to have a marketable skill. They want to raise a family. They want to enter a profession that is always in demand. They want to work part-time and flexible hours. They want to have some control over their work life.

Some new graduates like the elasticity of moving around the USA and living in different cities. It is more difficult for physicians to uproot and re-establish a practice in a new place unless they are part of a hospital or corporate chain. For example, *Kaiser Hospital System* or on the West Coast, *Catholic Healthcare West.*

I have met some nurses who go to school just for the medical knowledge. They then decide whether or not they want to pursue a career as a medical doctor. All in all, it all boils down to the personality and what his/her goals are in life. Some people like the independence of being their own bosses.

One has to know themselves. If one is the type of person who likes the freedom of being their own boss, pursue studies more in depth, and have the deep calling to assist people at the level of a doctor—then by all means put in the time, energy, money and rigorous self-discipline in order to go to medical school.

14. Why do they keep on saying that there is a shortage of nurses?

The infamous "they" keep on saying there is a shortage of nurses because there *is* a shortage of nurses. It is difficult for hospitals to fill vacant posts with qualified trained professionals 24/7. Health care is becoming more and more specialized. Not every nurse has the stamina and/or interest in the *Emergency Room* where he/she is constantly bombarded with continuous tragedies. Not every nurse has an interest in working with transplant patients or intensive care units. Not every nurse wants to work in psychiatry, pediatrics or the numerous other specialties. Not every nurse wants to work nights, weekends, or holidays.

Nurses by nature are very idealistic. However, to always be asked and expected to work overtime takes its toil on the nurse. Many experience burn-out at the day to day grind of the tremendous responsibility of taking care of sick, needy people on a daily basis. In order to preserve their own sanity and well-being, they gradually filter to less stressful and demanding work environments.

15. Isn't nursing very responsible work?

Yes, it is very conscientious and accountable work. At times it is very rewarding and satisfying. Nothing in life that is worthwhile doesn't have its' pros and cons. Remember the nurse is answerable for the care of patients. She has to be meticulous in delegating what she cannot do to LPN's or nursing assistants. She has to follow up with families, the institution where she is employed, the doctors, the administration and other outside agencies. She has to be all things to all people and keep her cool on top of that. Whew!

16. I can't stand the sight of blood. Do you think I should enroll in nursing school?

I say, "Fake it 'till you make it". In other words, that depends entirely on you and how badly you want the education. If you really have super-serious issues with it, then perhaps another career path would suit you better. If you can somehow stomach getting through nursing school and passing boards, you can enter some aspect of health care that doesn't require the daily viewing of blood.

17. Will they let me work as a nurse without a license?

No, they will not let you work as a nurse without a license. Once again, everything varies from state to state and facility to facility. Some places allow new grads to work as *graduate nurses* with the intention that they will pass their boards when they take them. But, in general, the answer is no, no, no. Passing medications and other skilled procedures require a license.

18. What part of the country can I make the best money as a nurse?

As addressed previously; it's location-location-location. Usually the larger urban areas pay more. New York and California pay more but as noted previously, they also have a higher cost of living. Check with a reputable career search engine to see what the average salary is in different parts of the USA.

19. Suppose I don't want to work nights and week-ends when I graduate. Will I be forced to do that once I am hired as a new graduate in a hospital?

Once again, that all depends on you and what you want to do once you graduate. In general, if the hospital needs a night nurse and you need the experience then one must do what one must do in order to get where one needs to go. Look at it as a win-win situation. You get a job, you get experience and the hospital gets a night-nurse. Usually there is no way around it unless you marry the *Chairman of the Board* or the *Head of the Department*.

20. Who was Florence Nightingale?

Florence Nightingale (1820-1910) was am English nurse during the Crimean War. She is considered the founder of modern nursing.

21. Who was Clara Barton?

Clara Barton (1821-1912) was an American Philanthropist. She was an organizer of the *American Red Cross.*

22. I heard that doctors are hard to get along with. Is that true?

That is not a simple question to answer. It is even more difficult to give you a straight reply. Just remember, doctors are people too. They are under a lot of pressure. There are so many conflicting news reports about questionable treatments; prescription medications; missed diagnoses; faulty diagnoses; botched surgeries; poor bedside manners; the list goes on and on. Ad nauseum. Remember, we live in a dysfunctional health care system. It is a political issue as well as a public health concern.

It is complex for them not to be defensive because the public expects perfection and healing from them. I once overheard a comment from a physician on why doctors are so rude, fearful and self-protective all the time. "We are molded as children to study hard so we can get into a good college so we can get into a good med school. Then once we are in a good medical school, we are then anxious that we won't get into a good intern/residency program. Once we are done with the internship/residency requirements in our specialty; we are then terrified that we cannot get a practice off the ground. Once we do get a practice off the ground; then we are afraid of being sued. Our whole life, up to this point revolves around getting our M.D. and then being sole practitioners. Then, that is when all of our problems really start. Now we are forced to deal with the sobering realities of the twisted business climate of health care, in short, finally getting paid. And insurance companies are getting leaner and meaner all the time. It is a vicious cycle. A lot of my colleagues wish they entered another field. The system does not support what is best for the patient."

With that statement in mind, it is no small wonder why doctors are not happy campers. Is there a solution for this? In Maryland, there are laws about working in a civil working environment. More importantly, I believe that honest communication with the medical staff that is nurturing and supportive is the best way to vent the frustrations that are inherent in any business climate. Negativity breeds negativity. Positivity breeds positivity. Enough said.

Some individuals, by nature are nicer than others. Doctors, nurses, and other health care professionals are people like other people. Just people. They are only folks. So to answer your question, I would venture to say that some doctors, like some people are more problematic to get along with than others. But, those few don't necessarily make up the whole. For the most part, in general, doctors are cautious and reserved in their day to day interactions. Paranoid? Maybe? It is delicate. It is intricate. It is just the way it is. I am sure glad I never went to medical school myself, personally speaking.

23. Is there scholarship money available to go to nursing school?

Yes, absolutely and without a doubt, there is tons of money out there just waiting for you to claim and go to school. Check with the *Student Loan Department* of the school where you are planning to attend. Also the federal government has money available. Check the Internet. (I would proceed with utmost caution about locking into anything on the Internet unless you are certain of the source. There are a lot of scammers out there in cyberspace) Go to the public library. Ask the librarian for grant information. Changing your life requires a lot of legwork but it is worth it in the long run. See which grants you may be qualified for. Then apply-apply-apply. Don't give up if you get rejected the first couple of times. Keep your eye on the prize! It is up to you to claim what is yours and what you are entitled to.

24. I heard that a new graduate has to work in a general hospital for a year before a nursing staffing agency will hire them. Is this true?

Once again, we get back to the one year hospital experience after graduation. Generally speaking, the answer is yes to this question. The agency sends only experienced nurses to job sites. A new graduate, without any hard core, solid, hands on experience generally doesn't function well. The agency has the obligation to the facility where they send their nurses that the nurse is qualified for the job at hand.

25. What is the difference between a two-year RN and a four-year RN? Is there really a difference when you are working together, you know, face to face, in the hospital, doing essentially the same job?

Once again, it all boils down to schooling, training, and education. Although two and four year RN's have the same boards after graduation; the same licensure exams; equal responsibilities when working on a floor situation or a clinical situation; the distinction is the length; the time; and the credits involved in the educational program of study. Nurses with a four-year degree generally get promoted faster. There are always exceptions to the rule and I have seen many confident two-year RN's be promoted quickly through the ranks. It all boils down to the character of the nurse.

26. Suppose I want to get my RN degree but I don't want to work as a nurse. Is there any industry that will hire me?

Once again, that depends on the individual nurse and what they have done in the past. Or it could be a question on how creatively the nurse has chosen to integrate the health care information to create their own job description. Question #6 and Question #12 delve into some possibilities with that. The bottom line is just because one is a nurse doesn't mean they have to work as one.

27. Will I ever get rich working as a nurse?

I kind of dabbled in that subject in Question #8. That all depends on what you decide to do with your money that you earn. If you are a single parent, supporting children, then you really do not have that much control on how to spend your money. It's usually spent before you cash your paycheck. Virtually, it's spent before you've earned it! But, if you trust a good investment strategist or have a unique business perspective on marketing your technical knowledge and expertise as a nurse, then you may just get lucky and strike it rich. Of course, you could hit the lottery.…

28. Aren't a lot of the drugs that they give in modern medicine unsafe?

Once again, a straightforward question deserves a complex answer. In short, that question cannot be answered minimally. How do you like that rhetorical response? I sound just like the politicians, don't I? But, on a more serious note … nothing that is ingested into the body temple is without risk. One could be allergic to some of the components in whole milk or eggs. One could be affected by red dye or gluten. One could be hypersensitive to Zinfandel wine … not all wine, but the grape used specifically in Zinfandel wine.

Different people may have special body chemistries. For whatever reasons, something ingested, inhaled, etc. may not agree with the person's body. For example, some people can get a bee sting and nothing earth-shattering happens to them. Yeah, the bite stings, but it is nothing that they have to call 911 for. Or, some people can get a bee sting and they do have to call 911 because of a severe allergic reaction.

Why can some people take penicillin and have no problems? Or why do some folks take penicillin and have a brutal allergic consequence? It's not that easy. I am no scientist, but there is some element in the bee sting or the penicillin that the individual body reacts to strongly and adversely. But, it is not everyone. It is just that people respond to unusual triggers in an adverse manner. However, if enough people keep on having harsh toxic reactions, then that particular drug is usually put under more scrutiny and/or pulled from the market altogether. (Alas, then the lawyers come in …)

Therein comes the responsibility of the nurse. The nurse monitors, observes and records all medications given to the patient under a doctor's prescription and plan of care. The RN is knowledgeable in pharmacology/medications. It is her job to know the side effects of the medications that he/she dispenses under a physician's direction. It is part of her job description to be aware of the side effects of all of the medications that she/he administers to the patient. It is her requirement to report any undesirable reactions to the doctor immediately.

So, to answer the question, "aren't a lot of drugs that they give in modern medicine unsafe?" There is utterly no concrete answer to that inquiry. Nothing that is ingested into the sacred body is without risk. The most important and imperative thing to note is: What is the medication? Check for allergies. Know the side effects of the medication(s). Call the pharmacist or the doctor about any concerns that you may have. That is the most simple/complex way I can respond to this question! Do your homework!

29. Do nurses need malpractice insurance?

Let's put it this way. In a society that loves to sue, nobody should be without malpractice insurance. Usually facilities have a "blanket policy" to cover nurses but it wouldn't hurt to have your own in addition to what the institution provides.

30. Can I work in a doctor's office as a nurse?

Of course you can! Yes-yes-yes! Many physicians' hire RN's for their private practice. Examples are plastic surgery offices, ambulatory care centers (one day in and out surgical centers) or other specialty areas. Some nurses work in allergy offices or pediatric offices. It's endless.

31. I want to work with underprivileged children. Do they have jobs for nurses?

It depends where and in what capacity. Do you want to work with underprivileged children in Third World Countries? Then join the Peace Corps. Do you want to work with them in the USA? If so, do you know how you want to work with them specifically?

There are many institutions with children who have severe emotional and/or psychiatric disabilities. Nurses are employed in these facilities. During the summer months there are camps for underprivileged children. Usually, they want you to have a year of general pediatric experience preferably in a general hospital. So, to answer your question, the answer is yes. However, you must research the different opportunities and what the special requirements are for the prospective employment.

32. What is a travel nurse?

A travel nurse is most times a Registered Nurse. (Although I have also heard of LPN's/LVN's with special skills doing travel nursing) Usually a travel RN takes contracts for a specific period of time outside of their own state. It could be for 4/8/13 weeks or possibly longer depending on the nurse and the facility. Sometimes a nurse may take a travel contract within their own state especially if it is a large state. For example, a nurse licensed in New York State who lives in Buffalo, NY may want to take a contract in New York City. Or a nurse who lives in Los Angeles may want to take a contract in San Francisco. Whatever!

Regardless of what state the nurse lives in, she/he must have a license in that state where she/he is taking the travel contract. (With the exceptions if it is a federal hospital, let's say a VA Hospital; she must hold a license in the USA. Doesn't matter what state she lives in) If the license is from a compact state, and the nurse is a permanent resident of one of the states included in the compact agreement, then it is not necessary to get another license. For example, an RN living in Maryland is allowed to work in about 20 states without obtaining another license in that state. She would be able to take a contract in Arizona, New Mexico, Utah, Texas, Wisconsin, Iowa, Delaware, etc. without obtaining new licensure in that state. (New states are always being added)

Usually, as stated previously, the contract is for 4, 8 or 13 weeks. The contract also may be extended if all parties are in agreement. The agency that the nurse is signed up with usually pays for travel, health insurance and housing. Some agencies are better than others, so one must do their due diligence in weeding out the better ones. A New York RN may want to work in California for the winter. So before the RN sets out of her door, she gets a job and a place to live when everything is arranged with an agency! She can keep her residence in her state and have the agency pay her rent while she is working in the state where she is traveling to. It's like having a summer and winter home and only paying for one!

Usually the hospitals are looking for specialty RN's such as ICU; ER; CCU; Labor & Delivery; PICU; NICU RN's, and every so often Psych. Sometimes they are also looking for Case Managers. Hospitals put their orders in for their needs. Agencies attempt to fill the needs from their talent pool. Once again, the agencies will only hire RN's with experience. No neophytes. Only pro's need apply!

The reason a nurse may elect to do a travel contract is varied. She/he may want to experience living in a different part of the country without the commitment of moving from his/her state permanently. A Manhattan RN may want to work in sunny Florida for the winter. It does get cold in the winter up North! Some nurses like the travel nursing for the variety. It is a wonderful way to explore the many fabulous places in the USA and live and work there temporarily to see if they resonate with that part of the country. Some nurses want to get away from their families, their husbands especially!

Travel nurse salaries are usually higher because of the "inconvenience and stress of not being in your home" on a daily basis. Many nurses elect to work six months out of the year and do other things the rest of the year. But, all of the travel nurses have one thing in common—experience. Travel nursing can be rewarding and fun!

33. The nurses in my state are always threatening to go on strike. Why?

Another brilliant question that only deserves a multi-faceted complex answer. In other words, that is not an easy question to answer. Nurses go on strike for several reasons. Forced overtime, sub-standard and dangerous nurse-patient ratios, better benefits and improved wages are usually the main reasons.

Because there is such a shortage of nurses coupled with the fact that many health care establishments have been forced to trim their budgets considerably, the staff nurse is forced into more and more accountability. The nurses just don't have enough people to assign the heavy patient loads to. It is highly responsible work to take care of ill people. Dysfunctional breeds dysfunctional. For example, a nurse cannot physically take care of patients; perform the necessary reams of documentation; pass medications; regulate intravenous lines; contact physicians and then be expected to wash the windows, scrub the floors and empty out the trash too …

Another reason is forced overtime. Suppose you are a nurse on a floor in a general hospital. You have worked all day long. You are looking forward to your evening to do whatever. Susie Q calls in sick for the evening shift. The administration may force the day nurse to work overtime to cover the evening shift. The day nurse is a single mother. She is now forced into a tight spot of not tending to her own family needs. How can she take care of them if she is not there?

The nurse is tired from the busyness of working the day shift. She is now required to work overtime. She's stressed and tired; she's worried about her kids so she/he is more prone to making errors. All kinds of mistakes. All in all, it builds a tension between the hospital administration and one of the most important citizens in the delivery of health care—the nurse! Face it, without nurses a hospital would be paralyzed. They would be unable to function. They could not deliver care to the community.

Needless to say, the situation is less than ideal if a professional nurse is overburdened; overworked; aggravated; frustrated; burnt-out and forced to work against his/her will because a hospital cannot fill its vacancies. It's a Catch-22 …

In some states like New York and California, a nurses' union and the hospital has a ratio of nurses per patient per union agreement. That sometimes does not stand though. Some other states also have nurses unions. All in all, the system as it stands now is less than perfect. In the perfect world … So what happens is nurses go on strike or quit because it is nerve-wracking on the human being taking care of sick patients. An *oxymoron* so to speak. I know that this response barely scratches the surface of this deeply disturbing, complex, and mystifying matter of why nurses go on strike. In a nutshell, that is the reasons *why*, in general, nurses go on strike.

Nurses, universally, are idealistic and good-hearted. They are patient advocates but they don't have the time to spend with patients. Again, the *oxymoron* creeps into focus, once again. The nurses don't have the time because their other tasks have them spread too thin to spend quality time with their patients. Nurses, being only human themselves, get fed-up and move on to less taxing and volatile careers.

34. I want to work on a luxury liner. Are there any jobs for nurses on cruise ships?

Yes! People, do get sick on voyages. Everything from upset stomachs; broken bones; to heart attacks and strokes. You name it; it can happen aboard a ship in the middle of an ocean. Usually the nurses who are selected for these positions have a general medical-surgical background as well as ICU & ER experience. The more diverse and well-rounded the experience, the better the chance one has for landing one of these highly desirable positions. A background in general pediatrics is desirable if children are on board.

Contact the Human Resources Department of any of the major shipping lines. The best way to get started is by doing an internet search. Then prepare to jump through a lot of hoops to get processed and ready to go. Pack your suitcase!

35. I am interested in natural healing. Are there any jobs for nurses in that?

Another excellent question! In the perfect world we would love to be healed by nature and divine intervention. However, the reality of the corporate culture that we live in, in the USA, shows that pathology (sickness) pays. Bad health pays. There is more money in treating illnesses than in preventing them. That analysis is changing though as more and more savvy consumers of the health care system are attuned to the growing market of prevention and natural remedies.

Green tea; vitamins; herbs; massages; Reiki healing; acupuncture; chiropractic; colonics; meditation; crystals; the list goes on and on. The nurse must be up to date and informed about all of these disciplines. If a consumer/customer/client of the health care system is seeking "alternative treatment" and asks a nurse about a different healing, then it is up to the individual nurse to be at least being familiar with their premises, although careful not to endorse any particular mode of treatment. That way she can enlighten the patient in lay person's terms. In their talk, she then allows the client to come to their own conclusions about what they think that they would like to include in their healing/treatment regimen. Remember, healing is a highly personal issue. What may work for one may not work for all. She should also direct the patient/client to speak with their doctor about what they want included in their treatment program.

In some states, they have *Holistic Nurse Associations.* Some colleges and universities even offer a degree and a *Masters in Holistic Health.* Usually the nurse trained at this level is more of a consultant as opposed to sole practitioner.

Usually a nurse, in order to enter into any natural healing discipline, would need to further her basic RN credentials to more of an advanced practice. Some nurses go on to be licensed acupuncturists, herbalists or naturopathic doctors. I know a nurse who was also a chiropractor! It is not mandatory in order to do advanced practice as an alternative practitioner to be a nurse, but any health knowledge that assists the patient into wellness is always beneficial. The goal is the same. To assist the patient to the best possible state of health and well-being. More is discussed later in the book about this area.

36. I want to teach nurses. What kind of education will I need?

Good goal! One of the reasons why there is a shortage of nurses is because there is a lack of qualified instructors. Generally speaking, it all depends on the level that you decide to teach. Most usually, in order to teach RN's on a community college level or on a university level, one needs a *Masters Degree*. An RN with a *Bachelors Degree* and solid experience can sometimes supervise potential RN's and LPN's in the hospital rotation and setting as this is a must to meet the demands of the school.

A nurse with a *Bachelors of Science in Nursing* can teach LPN/LVN students and/or nursing assistants. Once again, this is not engraved in stone. It all depends on location, location, location. Some rural areas have a scarcity of qualified instructors. RN's with experience can teach also. We are all teachers anyway.

Some nurses get their *PH.D (Doctor of Nursing; a Doctorate Degree)*. They teach, do research, and write scholarly papers, or whatever one does with a *PH.D* in *Nursing*. They are more likely to be connected with a teaching college and/or university. Some are even directors in major hospitals.

In summary, a *Masters Degree* is the standard, but not necessarily the norm. Hospitals that have specialized departments require that the nurses have a *Masters* in a specialization in order to teach the nurses in that particular department. They work for *Staff Development* or *Clinical Development*. Examples would be *a Psychiatric Nurse Clinical Specialist; a Pediatric Nurse Specialist* or a *Maternal and Child Health Specialist*, etc. There are many other areas of expertise as health care gets more specific all the time. It is impossible to keep up with it. A *Geriatric-Psychiatric Nurse Specialist* is becoming quite popular also. But as I said before, trust me, sneeze and everything changes in healthcare in a heartbeat! www.nln.org is a website to learn more.

37. If I join the military, will they pay for nursing school?

Generally, yes. There are many rules and regulations to adhere to. Usually you must commit to a period of time after you graduate from an accredited school to serve in the military in order to fulfill the contract specifications. So if you plan to go this route, be sure you know what you are getting into. Contact your local *Armed Services Recruiter* for details. Army? Navy? Air Force?

38. What is Bariatrics?

Bariatrics is a branch of medicine that specializes distinctively in weight reduction. Obesity is a complex health concern which plagues the American public. When diet and exercise alone do not render weight control, then many people seek physicians who specialize in *Bariatrics.* Surgery may be indicated in severe cases. Intestinal bypass surgery; lipectomy, (surgical removal of fat) and liposuction are the most common surgical procedures.

39. Can I work in another country as a USA trained nurse?

Absolutely! We briefly discussed that in another question but I will go into a little more detail here. There are some nursing agencies in the USA who concentrate on sending and placing American nurses abroad. Some nurses have gone to the Middle East. With the international political climate as it stands now, one would really have to examine their motivations for working in politically unstable areas, especially in the Middle East.

Many nurses join the Peace Corps. They go to India, Nepal and other Third World Countries. The criteria for experience are different in each country but usually the rule is one year solid experience in a hospital doing floor nursing or other specialty. The agency will know all of the essentials and fine points to assist the nurse in pursuing this kind of opportunity and adventure. Get your passport ready!

40. Can you catch diseases from patients as a nurse?

Unfortunately, yes. However it is not the norm. Most nurses have strong immune systems that guard against disease. The fact remains that nurses are only human and their immune system may get run down. When anyone's immune system gets run down because of stress, weariness, or other pre-existing conditions, etc., it invites a host of germs to activate in the body. This in turn may manifest as disease.

Yearly TB (tuberculosis) screenings are mandatory and required for practicing nurses in any clinical setting. Unfortunately, TB is on the rise. Since and because nurses work in enclosed environments, nurses are exposed to coughing, sneezing and other airborne viruses and bacteria. They may or may not be harboring different respiratory germs that could be contagious to the nurse or anyone else who's immune system is under fire or delicate.

Although hand washing and scrupulous biological and hygienic measures are employed, the sad truth is that germs are not bullet-proof in modern medicine or anywhere else on the planet for that matter.

Many nurses are concerned about needle-sticks because of hepatitis or HIV. Hospitals have strict precautions to avoid these mishaps. Needle manufacturers are also sensitive to this fact. They are forever perfecting newer needles to combat and prevent needle-sticks from happening. In actuality, the incidence is rather low to obtain diseases from needle-sticks. (Or so, it has been conveyed to me, but once again, that can change in a heartbeat) But, remember, it can happen …

So, to answer your question, the answer is yes. In truth, who is to say that you will or will not catch something at a supermarket, in a subway, on a bus, in the dead of winter from someone who continuously coughs or sneezes germs in the air? Or go to a restaurant and catch a stomach virus? Or yada, yada, yada … who knows, ya' know? I am not minimizing this question, there are so many variables. Reality is that it does happen, and that is the bottom line. However, that is not the norm if one is meticulous. But, as they say, stuff happens!

41. I heard that nurses get *burnt-out* with nursing. Is that true?

Yes, that is true. It can and does happen in any profession. People plain and simply just get *burnt-out*. That is purely a universal phenomenon. The daily rigors of the nursing profession and its constant demands, physically and psychologically, can be very strenuous. That is why it is imperatively important to make sure that the nurse keeps a well-rounded life. It is crucial that he/she not neglect other facets of rest and relaxation in his/her life. Also, because a nurse is often in a position to make split second life-death decisions, it is always important to maintain a certain level of humor and philosophy about his or her own mortality.

42. I want to be a Head Nurse. Will they hire me right after graduation to do that?

Dream on. Most likely, no. Once again, and read my lips, the administration looks to hire only nurses with comprehension for that position as it requires a lot of communication skills and knowledge that can only come with hard core experience in the field.

Of course, there are always exceptions to the rule. Let's say you are an LPN who just became an RN. You have been working at the same nursing home for years while you were getting your RN. In this instance, since you are known to the organization, the management may indeed hire you for that slot since you have known experience with the facility.

Generally speaking, the Head Nurse has to have at least one year of solid clinical experience under her belt as an RN. Remember, there are always exceptions though.

43. What is the Director of Nursing?

The *Director of Nursing* is basically the *Chief Nurse,* the *Big Cheese Nurse,* in any given health care organization. He/she may be *Director* in a hospital, nursing home, psychiatric hospital, rehab facility, or any other establishment where there needs to be a *Director of Nursing Services.*

44. Is nursing school hard?

Semantics, semantics, semantics! It depends on what you mean by "hard". Nursing school requires diligent study habits. It requires discipline. It requires that you keep up with the work. If you do not keep up with the work in a regimented manner (unless you have a photographic memory) then it will become difficult to stay in a program of study. You will flunk out. You will have to take courses over again. It will be tough to pass boards and practice as an RN. In other words, if you think that you can just whiz thorough a program without applying yourself then you are dreaming. Nose to the grindstone. Study. It is as simple as that. But, to answer your question whether it is hard or not, it's harder if you want the education and you are not willing to do the work. Why set yourself up for failure and waste your time?

45. I am scared of someone dying on me in the hospital. How do I handle that?

Good question! It is truly heart-wrenching to deal with life-death decisions on a day to day basis. A lot of nurses take up sports or some type of aerobics program. A lot of them have families. A lot of them take up hobbies. I took up comedy as a hobby because I love it! In the health care community, "gallows humor" kind of takes over to help the health care team manage their own sorrow. If the day to day realities of death(s) become too much of a dilemma, then it would be wiser to go into another branch of nursing.

I do believe that all nurses should have this type of experience on his/her resume. I believe it is through death that we learn about life. Death is a personal issue. It brings up all kinds of profound emotional feelings. The loss is permanent. Grief does not have to be. It is very emotionally satisfying to assist the family, if there is one, in helping them to cope with their loved one's transition. The nurse plays an intimate and integral part in supporting the patient and their families manage their sorrow and grief during this time period.

A lot of patients don't have a family or they are estranged from their relations, so the health care team is their family connection. A lot of nurses enjoy and derive a meaningful sense of inner fulfillment by assisting terminally ill patients. Death can be in the elderly or the very young. In the most holistic sense, death has no age. The spirit of the person is eternal.

46. My mother was in the hospital. It seemed like it took forever for a nurse or anyone to come when she put on the call light. Why?

I am afraid to say that given the current health care atmosphere in this day and age, alas, that sounds like almost the rule. It doesn't have to be that way. It seems like medical/surgical nursing care is getting trickier to steer through in terms of getting any type of real satisfaction. Staffing shortages, sicker patients, a nurse's time has to be prioritized and divided up accordingly.

I would suggest, for future reference that you take it up with the Head Nurse or the shift charge nurse. Address your concerns to them directly. Also, when patients leave a hospital, they are usually given a customer satisfaction survey. Believe it or not, they are read by the powers that be. This is an excellent way to air out any negative experiences with the facility. Of course, positive feedback is also welcomed!

47. Will I get good benefits as a nurse?

Organizations/institutions are very competitive in attracting qualified nurses. Depending how the nurse chooses to work for the facility, the usual health, dental, life, 401K (or some other retirement package) is offered usually in a "cafeteria style" offering. In other words, you choose the plan that is a better fit for you with the options that they give you. Vacation days, sick days, personal leave days, jury duty days, bereavement pay, life insurance plans are most commonly included in the packet. Most institutions also offer tuition reimbursement.

Some hospitals/businesses/employers are more affluent than others. They have more flexibility in choices for benefit packages. Ultimately, it is up to the sole nurse and what specifically the needs are for her present commitments. So, to get back to the original question, "will I receive good benefits as a nurse?" the answer generally is yes. Remember, it does depend on what you need specifically for you or your family.

48. My neighbor is a nurse in a hospital. She complains that she always has to take classes. She says that she doesn't get any more money for constantly taking all of these classes that her employers say will "upgrade her skills". How come?

Most hospitals are becoming more increasingly specialized. Specialization is the new specialty in health care. If she works in a unit where new knowledge and expertise are continuously being added to keep up with the changes in the field, like ICU's; CCU's; ER's; etc, then in order to keep in job she must do what her employer asks of her.

By and large, there is always something new in any specialty in modern medicine on any given day. It is endless. It could be equipment changes, medication changes, documentation updates, computer charting, federal/state revisions; the list goes on and on. When I taught my nurse's aides, I always told them, "That's the way it is today. This second. This minute. But sneeze and I guarantee that something will change in health care. That is why it is important to know the principles and basics because with all of the changes, I guarantee you, if you know the basics and have a solid foundation when something changes, you will always know what to do. In other words, remember the basics."

49. I heard that a lot of people die in hospitals because of infections they caught there. Is that true?

In the USA today, there is a reported 93-100,000 hospital related deaths each year because of secondary hospital acquired infections. The number changes all the time and it is dependent on what source the information comes from. Generally speaking though, usually the person who has a weakened immune system is more at risk to hospital acquired infections. One of the latest threats is **MRSA**. There is much literature and information published on this currently.

50. What is the average starting salary for an RN nurse right out of nursing school?

Once again, that depends on Location,-Location-Location! Region-Region-Region! City-City-City! Roughly speaking and I mean roughly, a brand new nurse starting out can expect to earn between $35-$48,000 per year. In some areas, especially larger urban areas and in some hospitals (especially large university or university affiliated hospitals), that number may jump to as high as $56,000 to $60,000/yr. starting salary. Remember, nothing is written in stone.

Let me repeat, read my lips, getting the Magic Number of one full-year of full-time experience in a general hospital, as a staff nurse, is the golden digit in making yourself more appealing in other health care specialties!

51. Suppose I don't want to work everyday. Can I work part-time as a nurse?

Yes, remember, as new graduate, in order to gain experience and expertise, employers are usually looking to hire a full-time nurse for the first year. If, of course, a nurse decides to stay full-time after that commitment, then by all means that is fine also as long is everyone is in agreement. After that you may be able to negotiate a win-win arrangement that is mutually beneficial to both parties. The employer has a nurse that is knowledgeable and the nurse has employment.

When everyone is happy then everyone is happy. Remember, rules are different in different places, so look at this as just a guide and not an absolute!

52. I heard that there are a lot of rules and regulations that I have to follow as a nurse. Is that true?

Yes, you heard correctly. That is supreme! Health care policies, legislation, and laws change very rapidly in medicine. Taking care of the public is a responsible job. Nurses and other health care associates must be in compliance with federal and state laws in order to keep their doors open and serve the community.

53. How come I always see want-ads for nurses?

Once again, as described in Question #14, hospitals must run a business 24/7. It is not easy to staff qualified people in specialty areas. For instance, a psychiatric nurse would not be qualified, nor would she feel equipped to work in the *Newborn Intensive Care Unit* with tiny premature infants.

The nurse would have to have be trained and oriented to the specific equipment in a *Newborn Intensive Care Unit*. Monitors, IV pumps, and other special care equipment require background knowledge in order to insure quality and safe patient care. Specialized observations that indicate a changing patient status are also unique in taking care of critically ill infants. Conversely, a *NICU* nurse may feel awkward and inexperienced in dealing with very ill psychiatric patients with their special needs and medications. The newborn nurse is more equipped also, to assist parents in coping with an infant who is critically ill.

54. What is "virtual recruiting"?

Virtual recruiting is basically like a "chat room" except that you "chat live" with nurse recruiters. These are usually scheduled events. You can go to a site like www.nurse.com and they will guide you to which hospitals are participating with the dates and times. It is a wonderful way to connect with prospective employers without leaving your living room. Remember, they are just as excited to meet with you as you are with them. Be sure that all of your "nursing paperwork" is handy as you may have to refer to it on the spot.

Also, this is a great method to explore other hospitals in different parts of the country that you may be considering for your employment.

55. What is *Continuing Education Units*?

Some states, like California, require all nurses to take *Continuing Education Units* in order to renew their license in that state. It is usually a course that is informational and factual. Nurses may go to conferences; take one or two day courses in their community or elect to do their continuing education units at home. *The*

Board of Registered Nursing provides a number to individuals, hospitals, and other organizations so that when the nurse finishes the class she is then able to put the name of the class and the number on her license renewal application.

Examples of courses that would provide *Continuing Education Units* or more commonly known as *CEU's* would be Diabetic Care; Seizure Disorders; Nutrition; Addictive Behaviors; Poly-substance Abuse-Treatment; the list goes on as the specialties in medicine are endless. When I taught my *Health as Humor: Humor as Health Workshops* in California, I had a number through the state of California so that I could give nurses their *CEU's* for their license renewal.

56. What is an "Appeals Case Manager"?

Alas! And yet another area of expertise! Basically, it is an RN or even sometimes an LPN who goes over client records and other critical patient documents. He/she then brings her findings to whoever is employing her—be it the hospital, the state, or insurance company.

Sometimes there are overcharges; undercharges or mistaken charges in patient bills. The Appeals Case Manager Nurse then filters through all of the patient records and finds things that may or may not be disputed for payment purposes. Mostly, in this job, they are always looking for a nurse with excellent communication skills both oral and written. They are most likely going to hire an RN with an abundance of experience in many specialties of health care.

57. What is an *Esthetic(s)* nurse?

And yet another field … of the giant field of medicine … and nursing. An (*Aesthetics*) *Esthetics Nurse* works in cosmetic surgeon's offices or in beauty type-spas, usually under the blanket of a qualified Medical Doctor who is board certified. *Esthetics* in the purest and abstract sense of the word is the study of beauty. Hence, think beauty.

Nurses who enter this branch are usually trained by either the MD or some schools even offer certification in the field. The nurses are then able to give Botox injections, do dermal fillers and even laser off some skin problems in certain clients. Different states have different laws concerning this branch, but once a nurse is established in this specialty, it can be quite lucrative for her. www.aspsn.org is a website for further information specifics in this popular area.

58. What is a *Legal Nurse Case Reviewer?*

A *Legal Nurse Case Reviewer* usually works with law firms or other specialty groups such as pharmaceutical companies. They review individual cases; analyze and advise attorneys on any injuries and the level of patient disabilities as a result of those wrongs. Or, if indeed, their damage was a result of any medical errors.

Once again, usually the hiring employer wants nurses with lots and lots of understanding in different aspects of health care. *ICU; ER; CCU; Surgery, Labor and Delivery,* etc. This is very valuable experience. Some schools offer courses and certificates in this area of expertise. Remember, a basic RN degree/licensure is mandatory. Superior writing and verbal skills are necessary for these positions. Also, a well-rounded background in medicine is a plus. www.inccertified.org

Remember, we live in a lawyer-happy society. This is indeed an extremely detailed specialty. This also can be lucrative as a consultant.

59. What is a Red Cross Nurse?

The most holistic definition of a *Red Cross Nurse* is a nurse who may be paid or a volunteer nurse that goes out to disasters at a moment's notice. Red Cross Nurses have been around for almost a century. If a calamity strikes, like Hurricane Katrina, then they are deployed to go immediately. Usually these nurses have lots of experience and the strong desire to help people in catastrophic situations. They usually have critical care backgrounds and Emergency Care credentials and qualifications. They also may have solid mental health preparation too. Some may have bio-terrorism training.

60. What is a Diabetic Nurse Educator?

Ah, yes, and yet another specialization in health care that is oh so important! According to the American Diabetes Association, the definition of *Diabetic Self-Management Education* is defined as: "the ongoing process of facilitating the knowledge, skill and ability necessary for diabetes self-care. This process incorporates the needs, goals and life experiences of the person with diabetes and is guided by evidence based standards. The overall objectives of diabetes self-management education are to support informed decision—making, self-care behaviors, problem-solving and active collaboration with the health care team and to improve clinical outcomes, health status, and quality of life." *(National Standards for Diabetes Self-Management Education,* American Diabetes Association. Diabetes Care, Vol. 30, No. 6, June 2007)

Diabetic Educators can be RN's, podiatrists, clinical psychologists, occupational therapists, optometrists, pharmacists and/or other health care providers and associates who hold a professional license. (For specific licensure info go to www.ncbde.org) Certification in the field is not necessary but it does add more creditability to the nurse seeking to be a consultant in the field. She may be hired by long-term care centers, hospitals, clinics, and other health care organizations. It shows that a national standard has been met satisfactorily for knowledge of diabetes education. The RN may add the initials, CDE (Certified Diabetes Educator) after her RN. She is credentialed through the National Certification Board for Diabetes Educators.

Having diabetes is a serious health care issue. "Diabetes is a serious and costly health care problem in the United States. As the primary diagnosis for nearly 44 million home care visits, 17 million hospital days and 82 million days of nursing home care in 2002, diabetes is widespread in nursing practice and a serious public health care concern." (CME *Resource, January* 2008, *Vol.* 133, *No.5, p.* 47)

In addition, the American Diabetes Association (ADA) has declared: "It is time for all health care professionals to treat diabetes aggressively. It is also time for patients to take their diabetes with utmost seriousness. And, it is incumbent upon the health care system to provide the necessary resources for both to be successful. Compromise of acceptance of a disadvantageous and dangerous status quo in people with diabetes should not be tolerated any longer." (CME *Resource, January* 2008, *Vol.* 133, *No.* 5, *p.* 47)

61. What is a wound care nurse?

A wound care nurse is a nurse who specializes in taking care of wounds. A lot of times, for a lot of reasons, wounds do not heal quickly in certain health care populations and diagnoses. Many hospitals even have wound care clinics. Many of these nurses are employed in nursing homes and hospitals as part as a wound care team. Generally speaking, wounds are slow to heal in diabetic patients and people with cardiovascular problems. (Poor circulation of blood) Wounds may become infected and the person could become gravely ill as a result of wounds not healing.

The Wound, Ostomy, and Continence Nursing Certification Board (www.wocncb.org) is the board that certifies nurses as Wound Care Specialists. In a specialized society the nurses who are credentialed through this board ensures the public and consumers that they are experienced, knowledgeable, a health care advocate and educator. This may be a branch that nurses may want to enter. Some home health nurses are also certified.

62. What is an *"ostomy"* nurse?

An *"ostomy* is simply an artificial opening into" in medical terminology. Many people because of disease or trauma have to have a colostomy, ileostomy, or an opening into their urinary tract system. The needs are special with this and they have to change bags often, find the right fit for a bag, and find the right formula to help the bag stay in place. An *ostomy* nurse is specialized in working with patients who have this special need. She can be employed by nursing homes, hospitals, clinics, home health companies, and other organizations. For further information about this specialty/certification go to: www.wocncb.org.

63. What is an infection control nurse?

Basically, an infection control nurse is a nurse who specializes in infection control. Hospitals, nursing homes, state and federal health care agencies are all places which a nurse certified in this specialty may seek employment. She is considered an educator and is distinguished in this field by certification. Hospitals and nursing homes are breeding grounds for any type of new strains of microbes so she must be attuned to new research in the field. For more in depth information go to: www.cbic.org.

64. What do they mean by nursing staff ratios?

Basically, nursing staff ratios means the amount of nurses per patient/patients. The *CNA, California Nurses Association* as of January 2008 just released their new state mandated ratios. It is a shame that this has to be law, but it is. Otherwise, unsafe ratios can lead to unsafe practice because there are just not enough nurses to take care of ill patients, whether they are premature infants, newborns, children or adults. California leads the way in this forward motion of safer practice.

The Ratios are:

Intensive-Critical Care-1:2 (nurse per patient)

Neo-Natal Intensive Care: 1:2

Operating Room: 1:1

Post-Anesthetic Recovery: 1-2

Labor & Delivery: 1-2

Antepartum: 1:4 (before baby is born)

Postpartum Couplets: 1:4 (baby & mom)

Postpartum women only: 1:6

Pediatrics: 1:4

Emergency Room: 1:4

ICU patients in the ER: 1:2

Trauma patients in the ER: 1:1

Step Down* 1:3

Telemetry* 1:4

Medical/Surgical: 1:5

Other Specialty Care* 1:4

Psychiatric: 1:6

All ratios are minimums. Hospitals must increase staffing based on individual patient needs. So the saying goes; "So goes California, so goes the rest of the nation". For further information contact www.CalNurses.org

Most nurses are idealistic and want to give safe care. Everything is always an uphill climb. Enough said.

65. What is nursing informatics?

According to *Villa Julie College* located in Baltimore County, Maryland, they have a course called—*Information Technology in Nursing and Health Care.* In their website, www.vjc.edu their description of nursing informatics is: "Nursing informatics is a combination of computer science, information science, and nursing science. Nursing informatics assists in the management and processing of nursing data, information and knowledge in the practice of nursing and the delivery of health care. This course addresses how technology shapes nursing practice, nursing education and access to health care information and examines nursing informatics as an area of specialization."

66. What is a public health nurse?

A *Public Health Nurse* is simply a nurse who works with the public, hence a Public Health Nurse. His/her primary concern is protecting and safeguarding the public. She does this by talking to clients/patients at risk and reporting her findings to the appropriate channels.

The more formal explanation of what a Public Health Nurse does, according to the American Public Health Association (www.apha.org) is as follows: "Public health nurses integrate community involvement and knowledge about the entire population with personal, clinical understandings of the health and illness experiences of individuals and families within the population. They translate and articulate the health and illness experiences of diverse, often vulnerable individuals and families in the population to health planners and policy makers and assist members of the community to voice their problems and aspirations. Public health nurses are knowledgeable about multiple strategies for interventions from, those applicable to the entire population, to those for the family, and the individual. Public health nurses translate knowledge from the health and social sciences to individuals and population groups through targeted interventions, programs and advocacy." (For even more detail of the definition go to the above website)

Community diseases such as HIV, TB and the HPV are some of the things that public health nurses are involved with. Toxins, world health, diseases spread from other continents such as SARS, also fall under her domain. These are examples of some of the things that may fall into the realm of public health. The nurse plays an integral part in this specialty.

67. What is an occupational health nurse?

Basically, an occupational health nurse is an RN who works in a business and or/in employee health. She may work in a corporation, manufacturing plant, a construction company, or a hospital, etc. Sometimes she gives influenza shots and does emergency care. Again, we are going in to yet another specialty of health care.

According to the *American Board for Occupational Health Nurses, Inc.* or go to their website, www.abohn.org, occupational health nurses are more desirable with a certification in the field. Employers know when an RN is certified she is familiar with many laws and specific rules that govern this branch of health care.

According to the definition of the board, the definition is even more specific and it is sometimes called *Occupational Health Nursing Case Management.* "Occupational Health Nursing case management is the process of coordinating the individual employee's health care services to achieve optimal quality care delivered in a cost effective manner. The case manager establishes or qualifies a provider network, recommends treatment plans, monitors outcomes, and maintains strong communication with all the parties." (AAHON 1994)

So many positions in nursing overlap with each other and as you can see, this is most definitely a very distinguished and knowledgeable position. As corporations and businesses become more increasingly accountable for the workplace environment, the nurse in this position must know a lot of federal and state guidelines.

68. What is a school nurse?

In the simplest sense, a school nurse is a nurse, usually an RN who works in a school. I have even heard of some LPN's being a school nurse. With such diversity in education in today's world, this may indeed be very challenging for some nurses. School place violence, and sometimes children with multiple medical problems are mainstreamed in schools. Some school nurses give medications. Some work in special education schools. Some nurses do emergency care if the situation warrants immediate action and triages the child, if necessary to area hospitals. Some school nurses follow up with children who have perhaps had a lengthy illness or some other type of medical problem such as seizures. Some may even do health teaching. They can work in elementary, high schools or junior high schools. They may even spot out behavioral problems and respond to what the school's policy is in terms of reporting it to the appropriate agency.

It is not necessary for an RN to be credentialed beyond her basic education, but a lot of employers are more apt to hire a nurse with a certificate/credential in school nursing. For more information on school nursing credentialing, go to www.nbcsn.org

69. What is an oncology nurse?

An oncology nurse is a nurse who works with cancer patients. She may work with children, teenagers or adults. She may be employed in a children's specialty hospital, a general hospital, clinic, private doctor's office or other health care environment. She is taught chemotherapy techniques as well as the many types of cancer drugs on the market. This is a very specialized branch of nursing and definitely requires thorough knowledge and education beyond the basic RN. Many employers are requiring certification. For further information on oncology nursing go to www.oncc.org

70. What is an AIDS/HIV nurse?

An AIDS/HIV nurse is a nurse that works with AIDS patients. She may be in a clinic, inpatient hospital ward, in public health, or working directly with a physician. Some nurses work with pediatric AIDS patients. She usually has advanced knowledge about this world wide epidemic that virtually is in every country globally. And yet another specialty in the nursing field. A credentialing organization that specializes in AIDS/HIV is www.hancb.org.This website informs in depth what the nurses responsibilities are and what are the credentialing criteria.

71. What is an addictions nurse?

An addictions nurse is simply as nurse who works with addictive patients. She may work in a clinic; in a rehab hospital; in psychiatry; in general floor nursing; in an advanced practice; it is everywhere that addictive patients are found. I once worked in a Methadone Clinic in Manhattan for a summer on a travel contract. Usually the patient population had multiple medical and social problems. That is not to say that addiction does not cross into all levels and strata of society. Alcohol abuse crosses all social classes. Gambling can be an addiction. Sex can be an addiction.

People can become addictive to just about anything. Alcohol, caffeine, nicotine, heroin, prescription drugs, etc. can create problems with relationships and economic responsibilities. The person will forfeit just about anything in search of their drug. It causes criminal behavior, violent behavior, lost days at employment, vehicular accidents if one is overly intoxicated, and in short, it is a public health menace. Since it is such a huge problem in the USA, many nurses are needed in this field.

"The *International Nurses Society on Addictions* (www.intnsa.org) is a professional specialty organization for nurses who are committed to the prevention, intervention, treatment and management of substance abuse, misuse, and addictive disorders including: alcohol and other drug dependencies; nicotine dependencies; eating disorders; co-occurring disorders; and impulse control disorders, such as gambling and sex." (From the *International Nurses Society on Addictions* website)

72. What is a nurse case manager?

A nurse case manager, in the most straightforward definition, is a nurse that manages clients/patients/customers case for a specific health care purpose. She may work with workman's compensation cases, in occupational health, HIV/AIDS, home care, any governing body that would need her skilled services. She coordinates with insurance companies, managed care companies, the state, physician's, social workers, anyone who would be involved in the customer's case. She simply is the "go to" person when different governing entities need information on how a case is progressing and what the status of the case is.

Many colleges offer higher education in case management, sometimes it is offered as a Masters level course. Nurses can be certified in case management. You can go to www.ccmcertification.org to get more in depth knowledge about this field. Case management, according to this credentialing board is defined as: "… the collaborative process that assesses, plans, implements, coordinates, monitors, and evaluates the options and services required to meet the client's health and human service needs. It is characterized by advocacy, communication, and resource management and promotes quality cost effective interventions and outcomes."

73. What is a transplant nurse?

A transplant nurse is a nurse who specializes in transplants. She may work with children, adolescents or adults. Transplant information is specialized knowledge. She must know about a lot of the drugs used, especially the immunosuppressive drugs. She must know about the complications after the different surgeries. A transplant nurse may work as part of a team. Usually the nurse must have solid experience and the willingness to learn about cutting edge technology and new information in this field.

Organs that can be transplanted are hearts, livers, kidneys, corneas, bone, skin, pancreas, hands, intestinal organs, lungs, bone marrow, skin grafts, to name but a few. Indeed this is very specific work. The *American Board for Transplant Certification* offers a certificate in this specialty. Once again, if a nurse is truly interested in this field, it would be good if she had the certification. For more information on this area of expertise go to www.abtc.net.

Generally, hospitals that specialize in this area are located in the larger urban areas. They may or may not be affiliated with a university or teaching institution. Some hospitals have a reputation for being a good transplant hospital.

74. What is a nurse midwife?

Usually, a nurse-midwife is an advance practice nurse who delivers gynecological and midwifery care to generally healthy women. They must be certified and most have an advance practice degree such as masters in public health, nursing or midwifery. They can work in private offices, medical clinics and hospitals. They can deliver uncomplicated births in the hospital, in the home or at birthing centers. They usually work with young girls to women going through menopause. They are usually associated with a medical doctor so if there are complications in a pregnancy they can work as part of a team. Nurse-midwifes can prescribe medications in the US.

They can assist the new mother with prenatal care, delivery and aftercare of the new mother. Midwifery is one of the oldest professions. Women have been giving birth since the beginning of time so to say exactly when it emerged is a mute point. Many nurses like this field because they are working with generally a healthy population. For more information on this area go to www.accmidwife. org. Generally, a nurse would benefit greatly in this area by having solid labor and delivery experience in a general hospital.

75. What is a hyperbaric nurse?

A hyperbaric nurse is a specially trained nurse who works with hyperbaric oxygen. The field of hyperbaric medicine is specialty into its' own right. A simplistic definition of hyperbaric medicine is the medical use of oxygen that is higher than atmospheric pressure. A hyperbaric nurse that is certified is indeed yet another specialist in the field of nursing. The *Baromedical Nurses Association* will give information on how to get certified in this area. Their website is www.hyperbaricnurses.org. This discipline is definitely a career choice that requires specialized knowledge in addition to basic nursing school.

Hyperbaric medicine is used in the treatment of different diseases/infections such as carbon monoxide poisoning; gangrene; wounds that won't heal such as in diabetic or post-surgical wounds; certain forms of anemia; osteomyelitis (infection of the bone), decompression sickness (divers disease), infected skin grafts or flaps; radiation infections to tissue, etc. For more information in depth about certification contact the *National Board of Diving and Hyperbaric Medical Technology* or www.nbdhmt.org

76. What is a flight nurse?

A flight nurse is an air transport registered nurse. She may be in the military, or be employed by the military. She can work as part of a trauma team and go to disaster sites like a wildfire; earthquake; war zone or any other type of mishap. She may be in a helicopter or other type of airplane. She must be knowledgeable in emergency care; intensive care; coronary care; trauma; pediatrics, etc. Usually this is a demanding emotionally and physically. She may be the only trained professional transporting critically ill patients from one continent to the next; from one state to the next or city to city. Many private individuals may also hire a flight nurse so they can travel if they have certain medical needs.

A flight nurse usually needs a couple of different certifications in advanced life support and be thoroughly familiar with all types of medical life-sustaining equipment. Needless to say, she must be thoroughly confident in her abilities which only come with a solid foundation in experience. The flight nurse is certified through the *Board of Certification for Emergency Nursing*. Their website is www.ena.org. She may also be a member of *the Air & Surface Transport Nurses Association*. Their website is www.astna.org

77. What is an XRAY nurse?

A radiology or XRAY nurse is an RN who works in the XRAY department of a hospital. Everyone at one time or the other has had to have an XRAY of something. It is a diagnostic picture that physicians read and look at for anything irregular such as broken bones, etc. Sometimes, in order to get a better picture for a diagnosis, dye will be injected into the veins and a picture will be formed to outline any abnormalities.

XRAY nurses, sometimes called an *Interventional Radiology Nurse*, must have superior clinical skills and critical care skills. It is good if she also has pediatric and infant experience. Some of the larger institutions and hospitals hire pediatric radiology nurses as a specialty. Also, the nurse needs to know the different medical diagnoses and have knowledge of adult as well as geriatric nursing.

The field of radiology includes but is not limited to diagnostic imaging procedures such as ultrasound; nuclear medicine; computer tomography (CAT scan); and magnetic resonance (MRI). Interventional techniques in the XRAY department would be myelograms, arteriograms and venograms. The nurse in this department would have to know how to start IV's; sometimes give IV meds; assess patients constantly and work closely with the radiology team to insure that the patient is safe during procedures. She could also work specifically with adult and pediatric radiation oncology.

This area is definitely not for the faint of heart. Sometimes the nurses must wear a lead apron because of the constant exposure to radiation. She may be certified as a radiology nurse. The *American Association of Radiology Nurses* is the professional group. For further information on this area of expertise go to www. arna.net

78. What is a nurse anesthetist?

Generally speaking a nurse anesthetist is a nurse with special training who administers anesthesia to patients. A patient needing anesthesia could be in any age group. Infant, child, or adult. The nurse anesthetist usually has to have a bachelor's degree and/or masters. They usually require solid critical care experience, in either a surgical intensive care or medical intensive care. Any emergency care experience, including trauma nursing is good also. The schools are quite competitive and usually the nurses with the education and experience are accepted in this program. These highly trained nurses can work in the military, doctors' offices, dentists' offices, podiatrist or even plastic surgery offices. They can work as part of a group or be in solo practice. The laws are different in each state. Some work with baby doctors.

The *American Association of Nurse Anesthetists*, www.aana.com is the professional affiliation. Information is available to the public on these advance practice RN's as well as information for the consumer. Some have a big role in the military and in VA Hospitals. In order to practice, they must pass a national certification test.

79. What is a rehab nurse?

According to the *University of Virginia's Health System* website, their definition of a rehab nurse is: "A rehab nurse is a nurse who specializes in assisting persons with disabilities and chronic illness to obtain optimal function, health and adapt to an altered lifestyle. (Sometimes disease related or injury related) They assist patients in making their move towards independence by setting realistic goals and treatment plans. They work as part of a team, and often coordinate patient care and activities."

"They help to restore and maintain function and prevent complications. They provide patient and family education, counsel and perform case management. They serve as family advocates and participate in research that helps improve the practice of rehab. The rehab nurse can work in hospitals, inpatient rehab centers, long-term care facilities, community and home health settings, insurance companies, private practice, schools, and industrial centers." (www.healthsystem.virginia.edu) Sometimes the discipline in medicine is called *Physical Medicine or Rehab Medicine.*

And yet another specialty among specialties in the nursing field. As you can see, it is important that a nurse be further credentialed in a field after experience and further education. For more information on rehab nursing go to www.rehabnurse.org. Their membership organization is called the *Association for Rehabilitation Nurses.*

80. What is a poison control nurse?

A poison control nurse is a highly specialized nurse who takes calls from people who think they are the victim of being poisoned or from people calling about a child possibly being poisoned or other types of calls. Her job is to triage, assess, counsel, educate, and do follow up calls to clients she has assisted and involve herself in the community. Usually, each state has a *Poison Control Center* and a 24/7—800# hotline for emergencies. Making that call can literally save lives. These centers provide emergency treatment advice, toxicology case management and poison prevention information.

An excellent and informative article about this discipline can be found at www.ohsu.edu/son/news/poison_catalyst.pdf. The author, Tonya Drayden, MSN, RN gives a riveting account of her day to day practice with this area of expertise. "This field is especially important in today's bioterrorism climate … the *Oregon Poison Control Center* is a team of specially trained registered nurses … the *OPC* staff utilizes their professional expertise as well as extensive collection of resources to assist in determining the appropriate treatment guidelines for poisoned patients … emergency medical physicians, who are also board certified in medical toxicology, provide medical backup support".

Entering this area would require critical care/emergency care and pediatric care experience. (Especially since 65% are child-related calls) The certification board for this area is www.aapcc.org.

81. What is a urology nurse?

A urology nurse is a registered nurse who is an expert guide that assists patients that have any concerns and/or problems with their urinary tract system. The urinary tract system consists of the bladder, the kidneys and the ureters, including the urethra in both male and female patients. They may work in doctors' offices, health clinics or specialty clinics. They also may work in hospitals that do specialized surgery. They may also take on the role of a consultant.

They can assist patients with different types of bags and/or equipment that may be necessary because of surgery and/or medical problems. Patients with prostate issues, bladder problems, warts, cystitis (inflammation of the bladder), kidneys stones, cancer, urinary incontinence, are some of the areas that they can assist clients with. This is especially important as there is usually a great deal of embarrassment and shame because for the most part, they are associated with the sexual organs.

For more information on this specialty, go to www.suna.org *The Society for Urologic Nurses and Associates* are the certifying board.

82. What is a transcultural nurse?

If I were to give a definition of what I thought a transcultural nurse is without looking it up anywhere, I would say that it is a nurse who studies that habits, and customs of a particular group of people different than her own. I would say that a certain culture may have a certain belief system that our civilization may not cling to. Such as, the removal of the clitoris in some African cultures in young girls and women. We may think it is absurd and cruel, and another society may deem it as a way of life. What we hold loyalty to; perhaps another tradition may totally disregard. Some societies have different opinions on death and dying while we try and sustain life to the end, wherever that place is for people. The list of differences goes on and on …

According to the *Transcultural Nursing Society's* mission statement, they define their purpose as;"to enhance the quality of culturally congruent, competent, and equitable care that results in improved health and well-being for people world-wide … culturally competent care can only occur when culture care values are known and serve as the foundation for meaningful care." (From their website)

In a conference PR statement, one of their objectives is to "uncover cultural care knowledge through hope and social justice in populations facing malaria, HIV, AIDS, and poverty". For more information on this association go to www. tcns.org I view this as an opportunity to discuss and exchange ideas of what can be done to help to combat some of the disease challenges that is wiping out various segments of the world population. Ah, for a better world …

83. What is a pain care nurse?

A pain care nurse is a registered nurse who specializes in pain management for patients. She may work in a general hospital, a university setting or other type of health care facility. She can work with the dying patient or the terminally ill. Pain management can be extremely personal for patients. A lot of nurses are biased when a patient continuously asks for pain medication. It is especially sensitive when it comes to infant and pediatric pain. A lot of nurses don't want to take the responsibility of giving patients pain meds all the time as she does not want the thought that she may have contributed to someone turning into an addict. Many of the larger universities and hospitals have specialized pain management clinics. Pain management is also a medical specialty.

In some hospitals, patients may manage their own pain if they are attached to an infusion pump that they can press to administer their own med. According to the University of Wisconsin, they describe a *Pain Resource Nurse* "as a registered nurse who functions as a resource and a change agent in disseminating infor-mation and interfacing with nurses, physicians, other health care providers and patients and families to facilitate quality pain management." www.cityofhope.org/ prc/pdf/UW%20PRN%20Role.pdf

Often, a nurse who works with cancer patients or a hospice nurse is certified in pain management. The *American Society for Pain Management Nursing* or www. ASPMN.org will give further information about this specialty including certifi-cation. Another resource for pain management is the *American Academy of Pain Management* or www.aapainmanage.org Specialties in nursing are the forte of the 21ˢᵗ. Century.

84. What is a dermatology nurse?

A dermatology nurse is a nurse who specializes in skin. She may work in a dermatology office with a medical doctor; with a dermatology cancer expert; in a dermatology clinic; in a hospital; or a health or medical spa. She may work with a plastic surgeon in teaching skin care techniques. The skin is oh so important and is the largest organ in the body. It acts as the first line of defense for any infection. It is important to protect the skin at all times. Rashes, sunburn, wounds, bites, birthmarks, acne, melanoma, the environment, etc. all affect the skin. Your general health is even reflected in your skin. Is it dry? Sweaty? Does it have a lot of age spots? Or does one have a glow? In our beauty conscious society, skin, and having good skin, is very important.

A dermatology nurse may assist with wound care knowledge and teach and educate about different diseases and ways to minimize any further damage. A lot of these RN's, especially the ones who work with wounds/or diseases of the skin or in a medical spa have higher education, usually that of a nurse practitioner. The *Dermatology Nurses Association* is the professional nurses' affiliation. www.dnanurse.org is their website for further information on certification and advanced practice specifics.

85. What is a lactation nurse specialist?

A lactation nurse is a nurse who has specialized knowledge in breastfeeding and human lactation. She is certified by the *International Board of Lactation Consultant Examiners*. The goal and mission of this worldwide organization is to promote breastfeeding as the worldwide cultural norm. They have lactation specialists in North and South America, Central America, Europe and Israel. The website for more information on this field is www.iblce.org.

"Clinical experience in this line is obtained in private practice OB, pediatric, family practice or midwifery office(s); public health departments, in the WIC programs (women, infant, children), hospitals, lactation services, birthing centers, postpartum units (after baby is born), mother-baby units, pediatric units, home health, prenatal and breastfeeding classes, home births (if legally allowed) and volunteer community support groups." (From the www.iblce.org website)

86. What is a Lamaze child-birth educator?

According to the *Lamaze Institute for Normal Birth*, the institute was started "to support initiatives that provide credible, relevant and useful information about normal birth to new and expectant parents and childbirth professionals ... forming the foundation for the *Lamaze Institute for Normal Birth,* there are six care practices that support normal birth and they are: labor begins on its own; freedom of movement in labor; continuous labor support; no routine interventions, spontaneous pushing in upright or gravity-neutral positions; no separation of mother and baby after birth, with unlimited opportunities in breastfeeding. Note the operative word here which is "normal."

Many RN's with OB/GYN/and/or Labor & Delivery experience are certified by the *Lamaze Institute.* In their website www.lamaze.org they will give the specifics on how an RN, (usually one with a bachelors or advanced practice) can get certified. They can work with nurse midwifes, doctors, clinics, etc. They can teach classes and work in a hospital setting. A lot of nurses love this field as they are instrumental in working with mothers and babies who, for the most part are healthy. *Lamaze International* is recognized around the world.

87. What is an orthopedic nurse?

An orthopedic nurse is a nurse that works with infants; children and adults who that are experiencing bone or musculoskeletal problems, (muscle+bone problems) They can be employed in specialty hospitals; general hospitals; extended-care facilities; home-health agencies; doctors offices; long-term care rehab centers and work for insurance companies. They can be certified by the *Orthopaedic Nurses Certification Board.* The web site is www.oncb.org. Some nurses love this field and wouldn't do any other type of nursing!

88. What is a forensic nurse?

A forensic nurse is an RN who works with victims of crime as well as law enforcement agencies, including lawyers. Unfortunately, this is fast becoming a specialty in the US because of the increase of violent crimes. According to *Nurseweek,* (a nursing magazine) their overview of what Forensic Nurses do is "Forensic nurses work with law enforcement officials as well as perpetuators and victims of crime. The specialty includes death investigations, correctional nurses, nurse attorneys, domestic violence specialists, human rights advocates and sexual assault nurse examiners. Duties may include collection of clinical evidence, determination of origin or circumstances of trauma, evaluation and alleviation of crime victims' injuries and rehab of criminals".

Places where they can be involved/employed are hospital emergency rooms, hospitals, correctional facilities, community health centers, psychiatric facilities, public health departments, law firms. The nurses can be certified through www. forensicnurse.org. For more information on this specialty, go to www.nurseweek. com/careers/forensic/html

89. What is a trauma nurse?

A trauma nurse is an RN who specializes in working with trauma victims. Some hospitals have specialized trauma units for adults and children alike. She must know emergency medical techniques because she/he is literally faced with all types of split-second decision making assessments that can plainly save a life right there and then. A lot of trauma nurses are in the war now because of their specialized abilities. Trauma nurses can be part of an air-transport team that brings patients out of the line of fire from accident scenes, or other disaster situations. Trauma nurses must totally be confident in their skills.

The trauma nurse usually has a background in critical care, intensive care and/or emergency room experience. This specialty is not for the faint of heart. It requires critical thinking and thorough knowledge. Gunshot wounds, car accidents and other types of mishaps are met on a day to day basis with this type of nursing. A trauma nurse may do flight nursing, work in an ER, or a specialized trauma unit which treats multiple types of injuries for both adults and children alike. A trauma nurse is certified by the *Board of Certification for Emergency Nurses* or contact www.ena.org for more specific information.

90. What is a geriatric nurse?

Simply, geriatric nursing is working with the elderly. The elderly population is increasing and more and more skilled nurses will be needed to fill these posts. Nurses who work with the elderly can work in day care centers, nursing homes, long-term care facilities, senior centers, assisted living, and home care. Many wealthy clients also hire private duty nurses to take care of their loved ones in their home. The elderly have special needs specific to their advancing years. Some seniors go on to live very long and productive lives without having to go to any type of senior care. Some keep on working because they can and they love it. So being a senior is definitely not a disease!

There are specialized areas of geriatric medicine such as Alzheimer's units, wings for dementia, geriatric psychiatry and other areas. Medicine is becoming increasingly so detailed that many universities and colleges offer *Geriatric Nurse Practitioner* degrees. A nurse who specializes in geriatrics can be a unit manager, be a Director of Nursing, or simply a staff nurse that works with the elderly. The *National Gerontological Nursing Association* is the official certifying board for this specialty. Their official website for more information is www.ngna.org. Some nurses may even get a clinical specialty in *Geriatric Nursing.*

91. What is a holistic nurse?

We discussed this in question #35, but here are some more facts about this discipline in particular. According to the *Nursing Spectrum* (nursing magazine) their definition of a holistic nurse is: "Involves all aspects of wellness and healing of a holistic nature; holism as being defined as the mind, body, spirit connection; that is treating the whole person not just a disease or symptom … the practice to being a holistic practitioner; (a massage therapist, acupuncturist), educator, trainer, general holistic nurse … they can work in holistic health and wellness centers, spas, health clubs, pain management centers and doctors offices. Some of these nurses even work with cancer doctors.

Nurses may be certified by the *American Holistic Nurses Certification Corporation.* Their website is www.ahncc.org. The *American Holistic Nurses Association* is the recognized membership organization. www.ahna.org. As we stand in this new century more and more people are seeking a more natural way of healing and these practitioners will certainly be on the cornerstone of consumers seeking alternate ways to heal themselves and prevent illnesses.

92. What is a vascular nurse?

When I think of what the vascular system is, I think heart and blood. Therefore I would say a vascular nurse is a nurse who specializes in these parts of the body. Heart problems, strokes, high blood pressure, cholesterol, blood clots, treatments and surgeries would all fall under this domain. Specifically, anything to do with the circulatory system would fall under this category. How many medications are there for lowering blood pressure or cholesterol? Lots, just watch the evening news.

The nurse is knowledgeable about the different treatments and surgical procedures. PVD or peripheral vascular disease could be fatal if not properly taken care of. If one is also a diabetic, and they get a wound, it could take forever to heal. Diagnoses such as aortic aneurysms, peripheral aneurysms, upper and lower extremity arterial disease, acute and chronic venous diseases, what kind of treatment and surgery is best for an embolus or a thrombus is some of the precise knowledge that nurses would need to understand in order to educate and take care of patients better. She would also need to know what the specific medications are for treating vascular diseases, such as clotting problems. What are the different lab values that are considered unsafe or safe?

The vascular nurse can work in a cardiac care unit; a specialized surgical care unit; in a doctor's office; a clinic; she can teach; get a clinical specialty or an advanced practice education. A website for this specialty is www.pcna.net. Another website is www.svnnet.org. This is the website for the *Society for Vascular Nursing*. So much data, so little time … a nurse may become certified in this area.

93. What is a mobile intensive care nurse?

A mobile intensive care nurse is a nurse that is trained to go to rural areas to assist patients who are critically ill. She may be in a helicopter or some type of aircraft, but the goal is essentially the same—to bring the critically ill patient to a larger facility where they can get the necessary life saving medical care. The nurse would have to have emergency room, critical care, newborn intensive care and or pediatric emergency and/or pediatric intensive care experience. In Australia, mobile teams would consists of a consultant or senior trainee in intensive care; a MD trained in anesthesia or emergency medicine, a critical care nurse, a paramedic or a *Royal Flying Doctor Service* nurse. Depending on what the medical crisis is, other specialists would also go along such as a surgeon or an obstetrician. www.mja. com.au/public/issues/171_11_061299/gilligan/gilligan.html

In the USA these nurses are usually certified at the state level. Usually the nurses are in larger urban settings. They function as part of a team. A newborn intensive care nurse may be certified in California to go as part of a team to a woman who is having critical issues with delivery of an infant. Nurses must have excellent judgment and assessment skills. Again, this is not a field that is for the faint of heart. This is very much another very precise field for the nurse who is skilled in trauma, emergency health and medicine. The state certification is called the *MICN* or *Mobile Intensive Care Nurse*.

94. What is a neonatal nurse?

A neonatal nurse is a nurse that works with newborns. She may work in a regular nursery, with moms and babies or in a *Newborn Intensive Care Unit*. Much of the basics of *NICU* are covered in question #7. The *National Certification for the Obstetric, Gynecological and Neonatal Nursing Specialties* has more specifics on this field. Basically, this is another field that has many different subspecialties. The official website for this field is www.nccnet.org.

95. What is a pediatric nurse?

A pediatric nurse is a nurse who works with children. Usually, the age group for this would be infancy to 18 years. She can work in a general children's ward; in a specialty unit such as pediatric oncology (cancer nursing); in a pediatric specialty hospital; a clinic; again, a pediatric nurse can be further subdivided into areas of expertise. When I worked at Hopkins in the mid-seventies, I worked for a year in *Pediatric Neurology and Neurosurgery.* We had all types of diagnoses that related to the brain and spinal cord. Seizure disorders; congenital birth defects especially spina-bifida, are some of the diagnoses we had on the unit.

Children's conditions can change very rapidly. The medications that are used; the dosages; etc. are some of the fine points of this specialty. Nurses must really love children and be willing to also be very education savvy, especially in teaching the parents about their child's condition. Children can be so rewarding to work with! As with many sub-specialties in medicine, pediatric nurses can go on to advance practice and work as *Pediatric Nurse Practitioners*. Websites for further information are www.pncb.org and www.oonc.org.

96. What is a foot care nurse?

We run with our feet; we walk with our feet; we talk on our feet; and when something goes wrong in our life; hopefully we land on our feet! Feet are important. We need our feet! So there is no small wonder that this too is an area of expertise! Foot care nurses assist patients with feet problems. Think if someone is diabetic or has a circulatory problem and they cut their feet and it doesn't heal? That can be fatal. The wound could not heal and infection could set in. The person could loose their ability to walk if foot care problems are not handled professionally. Period, end of statement. Feet are imperatively and utmost central to our daily existence.

The foot care nurse can work in a clinic, home health, a hospital, or act as a consultant. She has to know how to cut toenails; identify and make recommendations for foot care to specialists; in short, anything that has to do with the foot or feet. Rashes, funguses, ingrown toenails, trauma, plantar warts, are just some of the knowledge she is certified in. For further information on this specialty go to www.wocncb.org/footnail/

97. What is a developmental disabilities nurse?

A developmental disabilities nurse is a nurse who specializes in developmental disabilities. This is an important field now, especially with the increase of autism in the USA. There are some nursing agencies that specialize in this field. They send out nurses to make assessments in patients' homes. When you hear this word, think cerebral palsy; mental retardation; lead and mercury poisoning; Asperger's Syndrome; Downs Syndrome; fetal alcohol syndrome; children with AIDS; spinabifida; certain genetic birth-defects; etc. Basically a nurse who works with this works with the mental and physical handicaps of the client involved, including the family and outside resources.

The *Developmental Disabilities Nurses Association* is the main resource for this area of expertise. www.ddna.org. Another nursing organization for this area is www.specialneedsnurse.org or www.ddnursing.org. Nurses may become certified in this area also!

98. What is an emergency room nurse?

An emergency room nurse is a nurse who works in a hospital emergency room or perhaps an urgent care clinic. Auto accidents; poisoning; gunshot wounds; heart attacks; breathing problems; cardiac arrests; broken bones; child emergencies; psychiatric emergencies all fall under the day to day things that an ER nurse sees. An emergency room nurse has to be quick, confident and knowledgeable. She must be able to make split second assessments and act accordingly. Think of the TV show *ER!*

An urgent care nurse works in a clinic type atmosphere. Usually they are satellites of a hospital or independently owned. They see patients that need "urgent care" but don't necessarily have to go to a hospital emergency room. They are usually open about 12 hours a day. Many are staffed by nurse practitioners.

The *Emergency Nurses Association* or www.ena.org is the professional affiliation that certifies emergency room nurses. There is always a shortage of qualified emergency room nurses. Some of the nurses that I have worked with over the years would not work in any other branch of medicine because they love it so much. Again, it is not an area of medicine that is for the faint of heart. It is physically demanding and can be extremely rewarding. As you can see by this time in this book, being a nurse can mean so many ways to practice because of the increasing specialization of health care.

99. What is a gastroenterology nurse?

A gastroenterology nurse is a nurse who is knowledgeable and specializes in diseases of the esophagus; the stomach and the intestines, both large and small. When I think of the gastrointestinal system, I think of the mouth (ingestion and chewing); the esophagus (swallowing); the stomach; the small intestine and the large intestine and the colon. Think of all the things that can go wrong with this system. If someone has a stroke, they could have swallowing problems. If someone has a blockage of the intestines, this could be a medical emergency. In some diseases such as cancer, someone could have to have an ileostomy (opening into the ileum, a portion of the small intestine) or a colostomy (surgical opening into the colon because of blockage or disease) Gastroenterology or GI nurses can work with any age group; infants to adults of all ages.

If someone is having problems with ulcers; burning of the stomach; bleeding or blood in the stools, etc; they would have to have diagnostic tests. They would have to seek the expert specialist in this field in order to get a diagnosis. What is the treatment? Endoscopy is the field associated with this area. A lot of these nurses work in the hospital; in doctors' offices; in diagnostic treatment centers called ambulatory clinics. A child may ingest something and they would have to remove the object depending on where and what it is. Someone could have persistent vomiting problems or someone may need a biopsy to determine a cause for symptoms. These specialized nurses could work for manufacturing companies or other areas such as a clinical specialist in a hospital. (would require more education in addition to the RN) Nurses may get certified in this area. The *Society for Gastroenterology Nurses and Associates, Inc.* is a professional organization. For more information on certification go to www.cbgna.org. These nurses could also be involved in sales (equipment) or research.

100. What is a dialysis nurse?

A dialysis nurse or a nephrology nurse is a nurse who works with patients with kidney disease(s). Kidney disease can occur in any age group. A dialysis nurse may work in a dialysis center, a hospital or other type of facility. A dialysis nurse must know about equipment, especially dialysis machines. Dialysis is a way of filtering out wastes, salt and extra water from patients who have minimal or no kidney function at all. Sometimes people are on dialysis until a donor kidney can be found. For whatever medical reasons, sometimes a peritoneal dialysis has to be done if the dialysis can't be done through the bloodstream. (in peritoneal dialysis a catheter or tube is inserted into the abdomen for removal of wastes)

The main certifying board for dialysis nursing is www.bonent.org or the *Board of Nephrology Examiners and Technology.* The nurse who is skilled in this area may do corporate sales; work for the state or federal government; work with organ transplants; and various other educational possibilities. If she is working doing patient care, working with families is crucially important because of the chronic condition of having kidney (renal) disease.

101. What is a hospice nurse?

A hospice nurse is a nurse that specializes in working with the terminally ill. They work with other care professionals such as doctors; spiritual support services; families; social workers; or others involved in the patient's end-of-life care. Sometimes these nurses are part of a home health team. Sometimes they work in inpatient hospice centers. Their goal is to assist the patient and family (if there is one) to maintain the highest quality of life for the remaining time the patient has. They assist the family with grief counseling and act as a support system. They make sure the patient is pain free and comfortable. Hospice or end-of-life care nurses differ in their approach to nursing in that their entire focus is quality care for the terminally ill.

Palliative care is defined by the *Last Acts Task Force (1999)* as the "comprehensive management of the physical, psychological, social, spiritual, and existential needs of patients, particularly those with incurable, progressive illness. The goal of palliative care is to help them achieve the best quality of life through relief of suffering, control of symptoms, and restoration of functional capacity, while remaining sensitive to personal, cultural and religious values, beliefs and practices".

The professional association for this specialty is *Hospice and Palliative Nurses Association.* www.hpna.org is the official website. Some nurses may become a certified hospice nurse. They are certified by the *National Board for Certification of Hospice and Palliative Nurses.*

102. What is an infusion nurse?

An infusion nurse or sometimes called an intravenous therapy nurse (IV nurse), is an RN who specializes in giving IV's. She may work with all age groups and different types of diagnoses. She may give IV drugs, such as anticancer drugs in doctors' offices or in the home. Sometimes she may be part of a home health team. She goes to the home to administer a medicine, let's say an IV antibiotic in the convenience of a home setting. She may give blood products, IV nutrition, draw blood, and do other types of care that would require her to make expert judgment calls. She also may work in a hospital as part of a team. Sometimes she is also involved in research.

This RN has to be familiar with all types of equipment and other new data that is always changing in this field. New treatments; new types of therapies; how to monitor the patient for infections; infant IV's; pediatric IV's; adult IV's; possible emergency situations are all things that this nurse must be knowledgeable about. Usually, these nurses have a strong critical care or general medical-surgical background. Nurses often like this field because they can, for the most part work independently. A lot of times patients can go home sooner rather than stay in a hospital because they need IV infusions as part of their healing. They look at the skin around the IV site and change the dressings to make sure that the IV is intact and functioning smoothly.

Nurses may be certified, which is always recommended by the *Infusion Nurses Certification Corporation.* www.ins1.org is the website to get more information on this much needed specialty. The *Infusion Nurses Society* is the professional affiliation.

103. What is a neuroscience(s) nurse?

When I first got out of RN nursing school, I was employed at the *University of Maryland Hospital* in Baltimore. I worked in *Adult Neurology.* I worked with diverse diagnoses. I chose this specialty because I always found the brain the most fascinating system in the body because it controls the body. Stroke patients; seizure disorder patients; myasthenia gravis; multiple sclerosis; Parkinson's disease; are some of the patients that I worked with. When I think of seizure disorder patients, I recall all of the different types of seizures that I encountered in this specialty. Grand mal, Jacksonian, temporal lobe, focal seizures, post alcohol withdrawal are just some types of seizure disorders that I witnessed and assisted these patients in.

I also worked on a *Neurosurgical* floor and in a *Neurosurgical Intensive Care* unit at the *University of Maryland*. Diagnoses like brain tumors and the many types of them, i.e. neuroblastomas vs. a meningoma vs. a glioma are some types. Brain injury patients, neuro-trauma was also other types of diagnoses that I encountered. I also worked at *Johns Hopkins* in a *Pediatric Neurology and Neurosurgery* ward. There I encountered some babies that had congenital neurological problems; had hydrocephalus (too much water in the head) and they needed to be shunted. Sometimes I had patients that had spina-bifida or had a sac at the bottom of their spine that needed to be surgically removed. Some of the infants and children had seizure disorders. In a nutshell, neuroscience is a specialty among specialties. I found it fascinating and challenging.

The nurse who chooses to specialize in this area will find it very rewarding on some levels and very frustrating on other levels. But, as a whole, I enjoyed the time that I worked in these specialties. The knowledge that I gained was invaluable. It is not an easy field because of the constant frustration of dealing with chronic diseases or loss of mobility or other unknown factors that can happen. Patience and compassion is paramount in this field. The *American Association of Neuroscience Nursing* is the professional organization. Nurses may be certified through them. Their website is www.aann.org. Nurses may work as staff nurses; educators; clinical specialists; or even sell surgical supplies. Some work in clinics. *Neuro-Psych* is fast becoming yet another area of expertise, especially after brain-injured patients.

104. What is an operating room nurse?

An operating room nurse (OR nurse) or sometimes called a perioperative nurse is a highly trained nurse that works in the operating room of a hospital; day surgery center; a clinic; or sometimes directly in a physician's office. OR nurses can work in subspecialties of OR nursing such as neurosurgery; orthopedics; open heart; pediatrics; general surgery; ear, nose and throat; to name but a few of the subspecialties. These subspecialties are usually located in larger urban areas and in teaching hospitals. OR nurses are also critical during war time as many soldiers need emergency surgery to save their lives.

Generally, OR nurses have three basic functions. They are taught in all phases of OR nursing. Scrub nurse, circulating nurse and RN first assistant. (a first assistant helps the doctor directly during an actual operation). Sometimes nurses in this area later go on to become management consultants, surgical supplies salespeople or go into teaching or research. Needless to say this particular area requires a lot of detail and meticulousness, especially in emergency situations. The OR nurse must be calm and reassuring when dealing with any crisis that may erupt. Depending on the facility where the nurse is employed she may have to be the chief cook and bottle washer too.

OR nurses are generally paid a bit more because it is such specialized knowledge. Of course, this is a general rule but not the absolute. RN's in this field may be certified and it is recommended. The *Association of Perioperative Registered Nurses* is the professional affiliation. www.aorn.org is their website. www.cc-institute.org is the website for information on credentialing.

105. What is a medical-surgical nurse?

The med-surg nurse is the backbone, the meat and potatoes of nursing. They must know a lot about a lot. When you hear med-surg nurse, think of the average nurse in a hospital that takes care of patients with all types of problems. IV's; special equipment; diabetes; heart disease; transplants; orthopedics; appendectomies; strokes; and other diagnoses that may enter their domain while they take care of patients. They are usually employed by all hospitals. Generally, experience as a med-surg nurse for a year after graduation will open a lot more doors for specialties that a nurse may want to enter. This foundation provides a wonderful base of solid experience. Employers will look at this RN more favorably if she has this understanding. Although I have worked in pediatric med-surg floors, generally a med-surg nurse works with adults. Some more rural hospitals combine the two.

The *Academy of Medical Surgical Nurses* is the professional group. The *AMSN* also offers certification in this field. For further information go to www.medsurgnurse.org. Some med-surg nurses also work in clinics or in long-term care. They take care of patients who are ill enough to be in the hospital but not ill enough to be in an intensive care. When you think of med-surg nurses, think *General Hospital!*

106. What is an eye nurse?

An eye nurse or ophthalmic nurse is a nurse that assists patients who have eye problems. *Johns Hopkins Hospital* in Baltimore, Maryland has the world famous *Wilmer Eye Institute.* The primary age group is all ages. Infants, children and adults. Eye nurses may work with blind people; partially blind people or patients who have some kind of visual impairment. Cataract surgery; detached retina; diabetic retinopathy; glaucoma; injury to the eye, are some of the things she is expertly familiar with. The nurse may work-in outpatient eye surgeon's office and may be called to eye emergencies as part of a team. The nurse may work with families and or the patient doing teaching.

The *American Society of Ophthalmic Registered Nursing* is the professional group. RN's may be certified in this specialty. Eyes are important. Seeing is important. What would you do if you suddenly couldn't see anymore? Not a good thought. Seeing is something that most of us take for granted, like good health. Good health is paramount. The website for further information is www.asorn.org.

107. What is an ear, nose and throat nurse?

An otorhinolaryngology nurse, or sometimes referred to as a head and neck nurse, is exactly what it sounds like. See—ears, nose, and throat and one sees exactly what this area of nursing focuses on. When I worked at the *University of Maryland* in the 70's, I remember that they had a clinic and special instruments that they used in the OR. The area of medicine requires many years of specialized training for the specialist surgeon. Now think of all the things that can go wrong with the ears, nose and throat. Infants and kids can lodge foreign objects in their ears; surgery on the ears for different problems from hearing disabilities to the need for reconstructive surgery; babies are born with cleft lip and palates; someone may require that their "voicebox" be taken out because of cancer or other type of disease; people may be plagued with chronic sinus disorders; the list goes on.

Nurses are educators in this field. They may be employed by a clinic, doctor's office, or a med-surg unit. They could even work as an OR nurse with a physician who specializes in this area. They work with infants on up to the geriatric client. This is a particularly sensitive area of the body because it is exposed. Unfortunately, if for life-saving reasons, a patient needs to have surgery that could be viewed as disfiguring this would require that a lot of compassion from the health care team, especially the nurse. It is difficult for a patient to go in the world and be stared at by a gawking and sometimes cruel public. If the client is undergoing radiation, there could also be a lot of skin alterations that may be hard for some people to look at. The best approach for this would be to really work with the clients' self-esteem and try to get patient to involve in other activities.

Certification is available in this field for RN's. *The Society for Otorhinolaryngology and Head and Neck Nurses, Inc.* is the professional association. Their website is www.sohnnurse.com. Sometimes these nurses also make home visits or can work in a hospice setting for terminal patients.

108. What is a long-term care nurse?

A long-term nurse is an RN or LPN that works with patients in nursing homes; in a special wing of a hospital; assisted living facilities; group geriatric homes; or retirement homes. Or sometimes they can work in a nursing home in a specialized unit that caters to patients that may need mechanical ventilation but may not be sick enough to stay in the hospital. When I worked as a psych RN for a long-term facility, we had many patients with psychiatric illnesses. We had a lot of HIV/AIDS patients in varying end stages of their disease. We had some patients who needed occupational and physical therapy for a couple of weeks. They may have had a stroke or some other type of illness that would require this specialized treatment. Some of the patients needed to be fed through a tube in their stomach. We had some quadriplegics; demented patients; patients with Alzheimer's; or sometimes patients who needed IV antibiotics for a couple of weeks. These patients usually didn't have a home situation that would enable them to receive this care at home.

What were surprising to me were the age groups. I saw patients as young as 20 to patients well into their 80's and 90's. A lot of patients were in their 40's and 50's.

The face of the industry/profession is definitely changing. When people think of long-term care they think old people or the elderly in wheelchairs or in bed. That is not the case nowadays. Nurses in this area usually have a more long-term relationship with the client. It's like a second home or family that these nurses enjoy. A lot of nurses like the family interactions (if the patient still has one) and the less frantic pace of the day to day happenings. The facility was also very much into the Activities Department. They would plan parties; bingo; speakers; birthdays; etc. for the residents. I used to run a morning group for the patients who chose to attend on current events. A lot of patients enjoyed this as this gave them an opportunity to participate in a group and a chance for them to get know one another. This helped with a lot of the isolation a patient sometimes feels in a new setting.

The *American Society for Long-Term Care Nurses* offer a certification in this area of expertise. They are located in Pennsylvania. Also, a lot of RN's want to work in these facilities as a *Director of Nursing*. The *National Association Directors of Nursing Administration/Long-Term Care* offer certification as Directors of Nursing. Their website is www.nadona.org. Specialty is paramount in health care today.

109. What is a home health nurse?

A home health nurse is a nurse that goes to patient homes. She may do assessments; supervise any nursing associates in the home; teach families; give IV infusions; change wound dressings; change catheters or whatever is necessary to keep the patient at an optimal level of functioning. Sometimes nurses go out after a baby is born or after a child is discharged from the hospital.

The *Visiting Nurse Association* is one of the oldest established nursing agencies in the USA. Patients do better in their recovery in their own home. There are lots and lots of home health agencies in the US. If possible, this is a lot more cost-effective for taking care of patients in their own home. A website that is of interest is www.vnaa.org. One of the pluses with this kind of nursing is the independence and flexibility that it allows the nurse. A drawback is the reams of paperwork and now the higher fuel prices. www.hhna.org is another website.

110. Where do I go from here?

Where one goes from here is entirely up to the individual. This guide is simply just that—a guide. Nursing is one of the most challenging professions that one can ever do but it can also be one of the most personally rewarding. As you can see, so many of the specialties overlap with one another. No matter what, the main function of the nurse in society is to help that person to their highest state of wellness in body, mind, and spirit. So if you want to work in the Peace Corps, then do it. If you want to work on a luxury liner, then do it. If you want to work in the emergency room, or do flight nursing, then do it. Be first class with whatever you do because it really doesn't matter what you do in the long run in life, just give it your all and be the best. That is all that is required.

111. How do I get started?

Start today! Call your local college. Get the applications. Attend open houses. Get the information. The time is NOW! It is a journey! Enjoy it!

Afterthought ...

Putting this book together was in a wonderful way very inspiring and healing for me. I did not realize that without the nurse in society, medicine could not exist. A nurse's knowledge and expertise is so very critical to the basic fabric of this society, any society. I honor the nurses that are actively engaged in the field. I honor the work that they do. I honor the patients I have served. I realize that as I write this, I sneezed and something else has changed in medicine. The only thing that is the constant is the patient(s). The patients who look to the nurse for the answer in their hour of need.

I believe that being a nurse is one of the best ways to serve the planet. I do believe that when you put people first then things will shift in the right direction. Hopefully, in the USA, we will get back to that point of putting people first, not bottom lines and corporate agendas taking precedence. Health care is a necessity, not a luxury. It is a right, not a privilege. So if you are thinking of becoming a nurse, then this book is a great starting point to get you thinking about different directions that you may take after the basic RN education. Thank you for purchasing this book! Namaste!

Micheline is available for speaking and media engagements. Contact her at:

Free_rx_now@yahoo.com

978-0-595-48852-0
0-595-48852-8

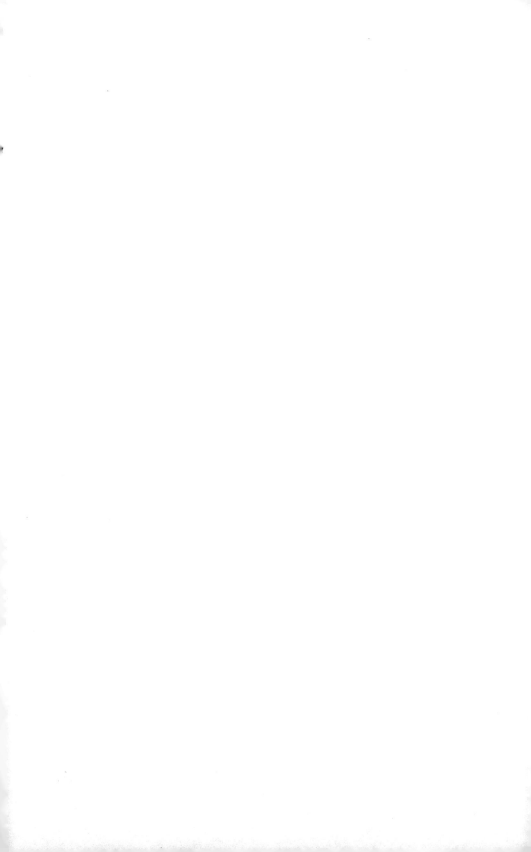

Printed in the United States
212052BV00003B/66/P

9 780595 488520